KETAMINE

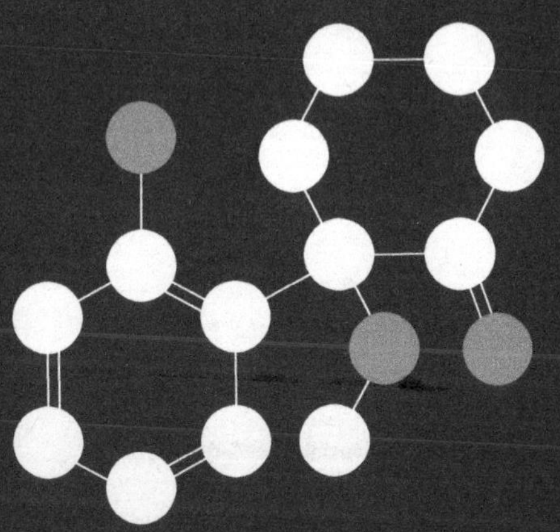

The MIT Press Essential Knowledge Series

A complete list of the titles in this series appears at the back of this book.

KETAMINE

BITA MOGHADDAM

The MIT Press | Cambridge, Massachusetts | London, England

This book was set in Chaparral Pro by New Best-set Typesetters Ltd. Printed and bound in the United States of America.

Library of Congress Cataloging-in-Publication Data

Names: Moghaddam, Bita, author.
Title: Ketamine / Bita Moghaddam.
Other titles: MIT Press essential knowledge series.
Description: Cambridge, Massachusetts : The MIT Press, [2021] | Series: MIT press essential knowledge series | Includes bibliographical references and index.
Identifiers: LCCN 2020010212 | ISBN 9780262542241 (paperback)
Subjects: MESH: Ketamine—therapeutic use | Ketamine—chemistry | Ketamine—pharmacology | Antidepressive Agents | Depressive Disorder—drug therapy
Classification: LCC RD86.K4 | NLM QV 81 | DDC 615.7/81—dc23
LC record available at https://lccn.loc.gov/2020010212

2

For Maman Shokooh

CONTENTS

Series Foreword ix
Preface xi

1 The Molecule Ketamine 1
2 Uses of Ketamine 17
3 Neuroscience of Ketamine 31
4 Ketamine as an Antidepressant 65
5 How Does Ketamine Produce Antidepressant Effects? 101
6 Safety Concerns with Ketamine and Esketamine 121
7 Where Do We Go from Here? 141

Acknowledgments 155
Glossary 157
Notes 161
Further Reading 177
Index 179

SERIES FOREWORD

The MIT Press Essential Knowledge series offers accessible, concise, beautifully produced pocket-size books on topics of current interest. Written by leading thinkers, the books in this series deliver expert overviews of subjects that range from the cultural and the historical to the scientific and the technical.

In today's era of instant information gratification, we have ready access to opinions, rationalizations, and superficial descriptions. Much harder to come by is the foundational knowledge that informs a principled understanding of the world. Essential Knowledge books fill that need. Synthesizing specialized subject matter for nonspecialists and engaging critical topics through fundamentals, each of these compact volumes offers readers a point of access to complex ideas.

PREFACE

On March 4, 2019, the Food and Drug Administration (FDA) approved ketamine for treatment of depression. This approval was touted by major news outlets as "the biggest advance for depression in years." The director of the National Institute of Mental Health, Joshua Gordon, enthusiastically tweeted about the approval, calling it "amazing news" and the first "truly novel drug in decades" for treatment of a major psychiatric illness. This was a remarkable ascent for a fifty-seven-year-old compound, a Vietnam-era combat anesthetic, and a 1980s club drug. The rush to approval was also unusual given the lack of strength of the scientific evidence, with only four small studies showing little efficacy versus placebo for treating depression.

Excitement has been followed by caution as concerns about unknown side effects of ketamine have been mounting. The FDA assigned a "black box" warning to ketamine, which is the most serious safety warning assigned to a drug by the agency. There are virtually no studies that have examined long-term effects of ketamine on the human brain. This is compounded by some reports of tolerance being developed to ketamine, which would necessitate administering higher doses of the drug to relieve depression.

Ketamine was touted as “the biggest advance for depression in years.”

Laboratory studies show that high doses may be toxic to brain cells, especially to a younger brain. Despite all the unknowns, clinical scientists are continuing efforts to get approval for the use of ketamine for suicide prevention in adolescents, as well as treatment of other illnesses such as PTSD.

This apparent haste reflects the stagnant state of biomedical research and the pharmaceutical industry in developing and marketing novel treatments for symptoms of brain illnesses such as depression and PTSD. The incidence of these conditions has been skyrocketing, whereas our drug treatment approaches have not improved for decades. Ketamine works differently than old antidepressant drugs like Prozac, which remain the standard way of treating depression. It acts on different brain proteins and has a rapid onset of effect. Ketamine therefore has the potential to revolutionize our understanding of the neuroscience of depression and how we could treat it more effectively. Even if emerging side effects dampen the current push to make ketamine available to patients, there remains excitement about this molecule as a scientific tool that can advance our understanding of depression.

This book aims to synthesize the scientific history and the biology of ketamine for a general audience. It will begin by providing an account of what led to the chemical synthesis of ketamine and the progression of its clinical and recreational use in the last six decades, leading to the discovery of its antidepressant effects. The status of the field after the discovery of the antidepressant properties of ketamine is further discussed in the context of making ketamine clinically accessible to patients and profitable. The book will then explain our current understanding of how ketamine affects brain function, including neuroscience theories that try to explain its antidepressant properties. It will end with some predictions about future directions in this field, regardless of the sustainability of ketamine as an antidepressant drug.

1

THE MOLECULE KETAMINE

Discovery of Ketamine

Ketamine was synthesized in 1962 by Calvin Stevens, a professor of organic chemistry at Wayne State University in Detroit, Michigan.[1] This discovery was not fortuitous. At the time, Calvin Stevens was working in collaboration with the Detroit-based drug company Parke-Davis to make derivatives of ketamine's parent compound, the hallucinogen phencyclidine (PCP, aka angel dust).

Unlike the deliberate synthesis of ketamine, PCP had been discovered in 1956 by somewhat of a fluke chemical reaction.[2] A chemist at Parke-Davis named Victor Maddox was attempting to make novel compounds that could penetrate the brain and hopefully have therapeutic effects. It is important to appreciate that the 1950s were the heyday of *neuropsychopharmcology*, a scientific field focused on developing and studying drugs that affect behavior in the service of treating symptoms of psychiatric disorders. In the earlier part of the century, there had been several serendipitous discoveries of drugs that influenced behavioral states, including drugs that caused sedation, improved mood, or had antipsychotic properties.

During World War II, efforts in this area of work had slowed down, but the postwar era saw flourishing pharmaceutical industries in Europe and North America, attracting talented chemists with close ties to academic medicine to synthesize more of these so-called psychoactive drugs. The modus operandi was to synthesize derivatives of existing compounds that could penetrate the brain and affect behavior or perception. These compounds were then quickly tested in animals and moved forward to human use. Nearly all of our current psychiatric drugs, including the most commonly used drugs to treat symptoms such as anxiety, depression, and psychosis, are the same as or me-too versions of drugs synthesized in that era.

An interesting example, relevant to the modern-day discovery of the antidepressant effects of ketamine, was the serendipitous discovery of our current antidepressant drugs. The drugs isoniazid and iproniazid were developed soon after the war for treatment of tuberculosis (TB) from leftover German rocket fuel (nitrazine). Doctors treating patients with TB noted euphoria and improvement of mood in some of them. This observation promoted these doctors to consider the potential usefulness of these drugs as *psychic energizers* and led them to test these compounds in a few psychiatric patients.[3] They observed a positive response and reported their success, establishing, for the first time, that it was possible for medication to improve depressive symptoms.

Their reported success, albeit in a few patients, emboldened researchers to test other novel and newly synthesized drugs for mood-altering clinical actions, including the discovery and marketing of the antidepressant effects of the so-called tricyclics. This initial group of drugs, synthesized by chemists at Geigy, based in Basel, Switzerland, included imipramine and clomipramine. As we will discuss later in chapter 3, these drugs remain in use for treating depression, as well as OCD (obsessive-compulsive disorder) and anxiety, under the brand names Tofranil and Anafranil. (Geigy merged with Ciba in 1971, forming Ciba-Geigy, one of the megapharmaceutical companies of that era. In 1996, Ciba-Geigy merged with Sandoz—which, interestingly, is the company at which Albert Hofmann worked when he synthesized LSD in 1943—forming the present-day megapharma company Novartis, with its headquarters in Basel.)

Researchers today look at the events of that era with both awe and horror: Awe because it took a short time, usually a few years, and little cost to go from synthesis of a compound in a chemistry lab to making a difference in patients' lives. These days, it could take many decades to

Euphoric effects of a TB drug showed that it was possible for medication to improve depressive symptoms.

move a new compound to the clinic. Worse, the clinical development cost of a drug is so astronomical that many potential targets never make it out of pharmaceutical company test labs.

Horror because the standards of safety testing, in both animals and humans, were astonishingly low. Drugs were briefly tested in a limited number of animals, usually without the careful long-term testing that often reveals toxic effects, preventing further investigation. (Aspirin or ibuprofen would likely not have made it to humans if they were discovered these days because their long-term high-dose effects in lab mice include ulcer and liver damage, which can be the kiss of death for compounds in development.) Moreover, once drugs were moved to human testing, there were no standards for placebo- or blind-controlled studies at multiple sites, which are currently the norm to get approval for human use of novel compounds by the FDA.

With this background, let's go back to the story of how PCP was discovered, which then led to the synthesis of ketamine. In the 1920s, chemists at Parke-Davis, similar to their competitors in other pharmaceutical companies, were playing with different approaches to make structural modifications to existing compounds with the goal of discovering novel psychoactive drugs. The field of synthetic chemistry has many *named* reactions or reagents, named after the chemist who discovered the chemical reaction

Researchers today look at the events of that era with both awe and horror.

or the usefulness of a reagent. The reagents are mixtures of substances that usually help with precise addition or removal of chemical moieties to a specific part of the molecule. Victor Maddox at Parke-Davis was using the so-called Grignard reagent (named after French chemist Francois Victor Grignard) to add moieties to a molecule (a-aminonitrile) that he hoped would have pain-relieving properties. What actually occurred in the chemical reaction was unexpected: instead of addition of a chemical bond, a substitution of another chemical bond happened (the nitrile in the parent molecule was substituted with an alkyl moiety from the reagent). This led to the unexpected synthesis of an entirely new class of compounds called arylcyclohexylamines, including phencyclidine (figure 1).[4]

PCP underwent some animal testing at Parke-Davis and was found to have unusual catalepsy-like effects.[5] What transpired next was a beautiful collaboration between academia and industry that, unfortunately, rarely happens now in the reality of academic-industry relationships. (These days, the nonscientific powers in pharmaceutical companies and academia, mostly guided by the influence of their legal teams, have made most interactions between the scientists in the two camps exceedingly difficult. Self-imposed guidelines and red tape make the process tumultuous, to the point that it is often not practical or worth one's time and effort to pursue any collaboration.)

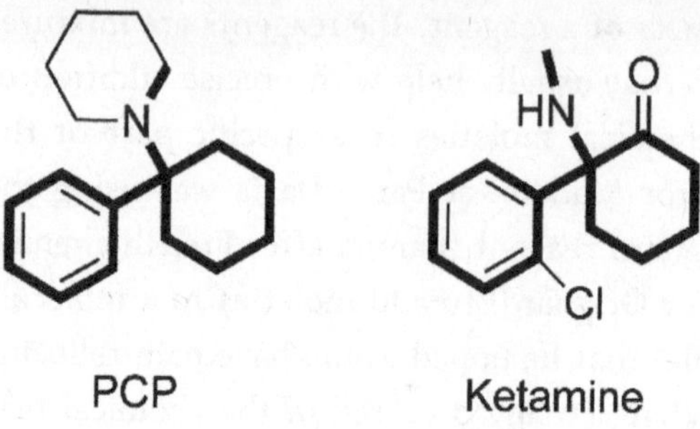

Figure 1 Chemical structures of PCP and ketamine. The common backbone of PCP and ketamine is depicted in bold.

Scientists at Parke-Davis, after the initial in-house animal testing of PCP, contacted a University of Michigan scientist, Edward F. Domino. Now a true legend in the PCP and ketamine field, Domino at the time was a young physician-scientist with a unique mix of expertise in clinical and basic neuropharmacology.[6]

Domino agreed to test PCP in laboratory animals and made the key observation that while in smaller mammals such as mice or cats, the drug produced catalepsy, in the rhesus monkey it produced a state of apparent tranquility and serenity. These effects were novel and unusual but suggested that PCP might be useful clinically as an anesthetic. Based on this observation, it was recommended that PCP be tested in humans, ultimately leading Parke-Davis to seek clinical approval for it as an anesthetic. The marketing name for PCP was Sernyl, based on

What transpired next was a beautiful collaboration between academia and industry that rarely happens now.

Domino's observation that it induced serenity in rhesus monkeys.

A critical property of PCP that made it potentially a superior anesthetic was the large dose safety margin, or *therapeutic index*. The fatal dose was over an order of magnitude higher than the dose that caused the apparent state of anesthesia, thus reducing the likelihood of accidental overdose. Moreover, PCP lacked the depressive effects on the respiratory and circulatory systems that are associated with commonly used anesthetics even today. This set PCP apart from all other anesthetics of the era, including opiates such as fentanyl and barbiturates such as thiopental, which became quickly fatal at high doses if respiratory support is not provided.

PCP went into clinical trial as an anesthetic in 1957 at Wayne State University in Detroit.[7] The drug proved to be safe and effective as an anesthetic, but in many patients it led to a postsurgical state of hallucinations, convulsions, and other behaviors that resembled symptoms of schizophrenia. Another physician at Wayne State at the time, Elliot Luby, took note of this and began to use PCP as a model of schizophrenia.[8] That model remains a widely used experimental tool in the laboratory.[9]

Because of these emerging side effects, PCP was not marketed further.[10] But its safety profile and unusual mode of eliciting anesthesia prompted Parke-Davis and its consultants to continue to develop safer versions of

PCP, ideally seeking a version that had similar anesthetic properties but was devoid of the lasting state of delirium.

A few years later, ketamine was one of the compounds synthesized as part of this effort in Calvin Stevens's chemistry lab at Wayne State University. Thus, the discovery of ketamine is the result of a concerted effort by the pharmaceutical company Parke-Davis and its academic collaborators to synthesize analogs of PCP.

Ketamine was tested at Parke-Davis and found to have similar but shorter-acting anesthetic properties as those in PCP. Domino was called on again to test the compound and led the first human trials with ketamine in 1964.[11] The studies found ketamine to be a safe and short-acting anesthetic with the added bonus of analgesic (pain-relieving) properties. Similar to PCP, ketamine caused a state of delirium and an unusual state of consciousness and dissociation from the environment. But this effect appeared to be less profound and shorter acting than was observed with PCP. This made ketamine clinically acceptable, leading to its approval for clinical use as an anesthetic by the FDA in 1970.

Mirror Images of Ketamine

One last interesting point about the molecule ketamine before we delve into its actions in the brain is that it is

Similar to PCP, ketamine caused a state of delirium and an unusual state of consciousness and dissociation from the environment.

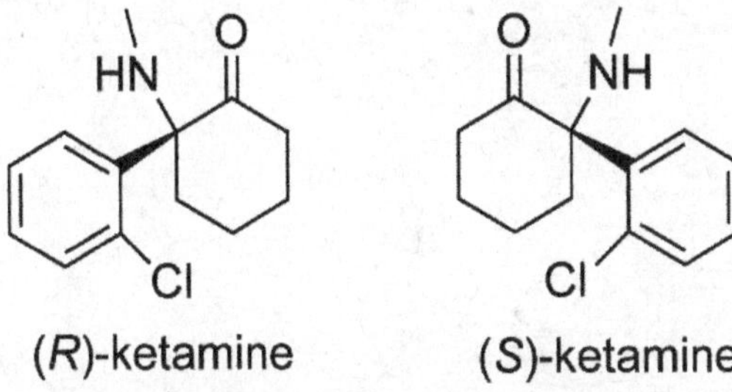

Figure 2 Mirror images of ketamine, showing the left- and right-handed versions of the molecule.

a *chiral compound*. That means that ketamine that is usually synthesized in the laboratory is actually a mix of two molecules, or two isomers, that are mirror images of each other. These molecules have the same atoms and the same general structure, but like left and right hands they are not superimposable. This is a fundamental property of some biological molecules, such as amino acids. The left-handed and right-handed versions of ketamine are shown in figure 2.

Many drugs have this property, but the effect of the different mirror images of the compound on the ultimate function of the molecule may not be different. In the case of ketamine, however, this difference is not trivial for two reasons. First, different mirror images of ketamine have different properties in the brain. For example, S-ketamine

Ketamine is a mix of two molecules that are mirror images of each other.

(esketamine) is more potent in causing psychotic symptoms and in producing anesthesia. Second, because esketamine and R-ketamine (arketamine) are technically considered different molecules than ketamine in the context of use-patent laws, the focus on obtaining FDA approval for use of one of the isomers has been a critical factor for profit considerations. We will discuss this further in chapter 6.

2

USES OF KETAMINE

Ketamine as a Military Anesthetic

The Vietnam War was raging in 1970 when ketamine entered the market as an anesthetic. This was shortly after the bloodiest year of the war in 1968 (over sixteen thousand American and allied soldiers killed and eighty-seven thousand wounded). The carnage continued in 1970 with over six thousand American servicemen and servicewomen killed and over fifty thousand wounded. Combat medics fought courageously to save the lives of the wounded, often working on an active battlefield, with the aim of treating and evacuating.

It is no surprise that ketamine quickly became useful as a battlefield anesthetic.[1] It had all the favorable characteristics: it had an excellent safety margin because it is rarely fatal, and it had a rapid onset of action, starting to work within a few minutes after administration. Ketamine also had the added benefit of temporarily relieving pain.[2] These characteristics made it an ideal anesthetic when time was of the essence and when there was no, or limited, access to resources usually available in surgical suites.

The commonly used anesthetics of the time, such as pentothal and other barbiturates, suppress respiratory and circulatory systems of the body and thus could quickly become fatal. Ketamine not only does not suppress these systems, but may mildly stimulate them. In addition, under ketamine, airway reflexes are preserved, and body temperature is not affected. This allows ketamine to be used safely as an anesthetic without access to ventilation and other equipment to monitor and rescue respiratory and circulatory functions.

Ketamine has remained an ideal anesthetic for emergency surgeries in field conditions, including in multiple military conflicts and war zones.[3]

Current Uses of Ketamine as an Anesthetic

Because of ketamine's short duration of action as an anesthetic and postanesthesia psychotic effects, it is less commonly used these days as a surgical anesthetic. But ketamine remains in use as a pediatric anesthetic, especially

Ketamine quickly became useful as a battlefield anesthetic in Vietnam because it was rarely fatal and had a rapid onset of action.

for minor surgical procedures, because it does not require intubation or other invasive procedures that may cause distress and complications in children.[4]

Ketamine's lack of effect on airway reflexes also makes it a valuable anesthetic in cases in which asthma or other chronic obstructive airway diseases may prevent intubation. This makes it useful in austere conditions for use by first responders when access to surgical anesthesia equipment is limited and/or if individuals being treated are under unknown cardiovascular distress or suffering from hypothermia.[5] Another reason ketamine administration is convenient for first-responders in disaster situations is that it can be administered intramuscularly, intravenously, and intranasally. Most recently, ketamine was used in the dramatic rescue of the young boys that were stranded in the Tham Luang cave with their soccer teammates and coach, with news outlets such as CNN touting the headline, "Boys Rescued from Thai Cave Were Sedated with Ketamine."[6]

Ketamine Remains a Popular Veterinary Anesthetic

Ketamine is commonly used for starting and maintaining anesthesia in veterinary medicine.[7] It is a popular anesthetic in this context because it is safe, effective, and has a rapid onset. Animals do not have to be intubated. The fact that ketamine is cheap is also an advantage. Ketamine can be used as a short-acting veterinary anesthesia in small animals, including cats and dogs. In larger animals, including horses, it is primarily used for induction of anesthesia.

Ketamine for Managing Pain

Low doses of ketamine have been used extensively for acute and chronic pain management.[8] This is a common *off-label use* of ketamine—that is, use for conditions not approved by the FDA. Ketamine has been used for postoperative pain management both alone and in conjunction with opiates to reduce their side effects, such as nausea and vomiting. Low doses of ketamine also increase the effectiveness of opiates in reducing pain. There is accumulating evidence to suggest that ketamine is useful for treating opiate-resistant cancer-related pain.[9]

Illicit Use of Ketamine

Reports of recreational use of ketamine to alter one's state of consciousness began to emerge in the late 1970s. It became a popular club drug in the 1980s and continues to be abused under the street names vitamin K, super K, special K, superacid, and cat Valium, to name a few.[10] At lower doses, ketamine produces a dissociative and depersonalization state sometimes referred to as K-land. This state is characterized by a sense of detachment from the physical body and external realities. Higher doses are associated with amnesia, more intense dissociations, paranoia, and hallucinations. This state is sometimes called a K-hole.

The combined amnestic and altered perceptual effects of ketamine contribute to its use as a date rape drug. Because of ketamine's rapid course of action, a victim may not realize that they have been drugged before they lose consciousness and may remember little about events immediately before they were exposed to ketamine.

Illicit use of ketamine has been on the rise in Southeast Asia, including China and Malaysia, with apparent high prevalence of use among adolescents.[11] In Hong Kong, its increased popularity as a club drug has been startling, with reportedly over 75 percent of people under age twenty-one having used it. The short-lasting effects of ketamine allow the user to experience a quick high during a lunch or recess break and return to work or school without the lingering effects that are associated with other drugs of abuse.

Ketamine's illicit use has been implicated in deaths resulting from drowning, traffic accidents, and suicides.[12] The fatal effects of ketamine are distinct from those of other illicit drug use, where the drug itself (such as is the case with opiates, alcohol, or cocaine) causes death because of its direct impact on disrupting the cardiovascular system. Ketamine kills acutely by putting the mind in an altered state. This state involves *dissociation* of the brain and brain-guided perceptions and actions from the immediate environment. How can this be fatal? It can prevent the brain from recalling and executing automatic or learned survival behaviors, such as instinctively not staying in cold water too long to prevent death by hypothermia.

Repeated use of ketamine can exacerbate its psychotic effects, induce seizures, and cause serious urinary tract pathologies, such as ulcerative cystitis.[13] The latter condition has been dubbed *the murderer of young bladders*. The incidence of this unpleasant condition, which can lead to lasting deterioration of renal function, has been on a dramatic rise in cities where ketamine is in common use.

A relatively rich underground literature has described individual experiences with ketamine. These include essays and interviews by D. M. Turner, who authored the book *The Essential Psychedelic Guide*. Turner died at the age of thirty-four by drowning in his bathtub under the influence of ketamine.

Ketamine as a Research Tool

This book is about ketamine's impact as an antidepressant, but to get to that discovery we need to first tell the story of how it got back to clinical experimentation in the early 1990s. Up to that point, licit use of ketamine had been limited to its approved role as an anesthetic and off-label use as an analgesic. The antidepressant chapter of ketamine's life, similar to its discovery, is also owed to PCP.

In the 1980s, two decades after PCP was synthesized and given to people, it was discovered that PCP disrupts the function of a specific brain receptor, the NMDA receptor.[14] This receptor is found throughout the brain and is usually activated by the neurotransmitter glutamate (we will discuss this in more detail in chapter 3). This discovery, complemented by Luby's observation that PCP produces a schizophrenia-like state in some individuals, inspired many researchers (the author included) to investigate the role of PCP and similar drugs on brain function as a means of gaining a better understanding of neuronal mechanisms that may have gone awry during schizophrenia.[15]

Schizophrenia is one of the most devastating brain disorders, and our approaches to treating it remain inadequate. Drugs used currently to treat schizophrenia have not changed much since the accidental discovery of the antipsychotic properties of chlorpromazine in 1950. Subsequent antipsychotic drugs have all been me-too drugs that are only effective in treating some symptoms of the illness in a subpopulation. These drugs also have profound side effects.

The antidepressant chapter of ketamine's life, similar to its discovery, is also owed to PCP.

In the 1990s, several investigators began to use PCP-based animal models with an appreciation of PCP's effect on the brain's NMDA receptors. These attempts led to the discovery of novel mechanisms and potential drugs for treating schizophrenia that had entirely different mechanisms of action than the traditional antipsychotics. These included studies from the author's lab, which at the time was at Yale, and those of Joseph Coyle at Harvard and Daniel Javitt from the Nathan S. Kline Institute for Psychiatric Research.[16]

One of the author's contemporaries at Yale was John Krystal, a young psychiatrist who was heading a clinical and research program focused on psychotic disorders at the Yale-affiliated West Haven VA Medical Center. Knowing firsthand about the limitations in the efficacy of the available antipsychotic drugs for his patients, he became interested in studying the applicability of translating some of the basic laboratory findings with the PCP model to humans. The general idea was to establish how a drug like PCP produces transient changes in behavior and brain activity in healthy human volunteers that resemble those of patients with schizophrenia. Doing so could inform us about potential brain systems that may be causing the aberrant symptoms of schizophrenia. More importantly, it could provide researchers with a model to test if drugs discovered to reverse the effects of PCP in animal models would do the same in humans.

Giving people PCP was out of the question because it was not approved by the FDA for human use. Ketamine, on the other hand, remained approved for human use as an anesthetic. John Krystal therefore set out to conduct the first placebo-controlled clinical trials in healthy volunteers to determine if subanesthetic doses of ketamine are similar to PCP in transiently modeling symptoms of schizophrenia in healthy individuals. The first results were published in 1994, showing that ketamine indeed produced a temporary change in cognition and behavior that resembles some aspects of schizophrenia.[17] In collaboration with his work, the author's lab shifted from working with PCP to studying the impact of ketamine on rodent brain and behavior, confirming some similarities with the PCP model.[18]

There were follow-up visits with the individuals who volunteered for the ketamine studies led by Krystal to ensure that no lasting adverse effects ensued. While the focus of ketamine trials had not been on mood or depressive disorders, some observations led the group to conclude that ketamine can be used safely and to suspect that ketamine might have mood-enhancing properties. The West Haven VA Medical Center had a strong mood disorder clinical presence, leading it to perform a limited proof-of-concept trial to test the impact of ketamine infusion in depressed patients. This study, published in

2000, was limited to only seven subjects, but it demonstrated, for the first time, a statistically significant rapid improvement of depressive symptoms.[19] Thus, the use of ketamine to model schizophrenia in the laboratory facilitated the discovery of its antidepressant effects. We will continue this story in chapter 5.

Use of ketamine to model schizophrenia in the laboratory facilitated the discovery of its antidepressant effects.

NEUROSCIENCE OF KETAMINE

A Few Basic Neuroscience Facts

Much of the excitement about the antidepressant effects of ketamine centers on its mechanism of action on the brain being different from traditional antidepressant drugs. In this chapter, some fundamental information about how the brain operates is reviewed before we delve into our knowledge of ketamine's effects on the brain.

The brain is essentially a communication machine. At a minimum, it must receive information from the environment, interpret that information in context, and generate a *response*. That response can be an action, a feeling, or something you are unaware of, such as regulating your heart rate. But it is often a combination of multiple responses.

The brain is essentially a communication machine. At a minimum, it must receive information from the environment, interpret that information in context, and generate a *response*.

Let's consider a simple example of one piece of information from the environment eliciting a response: you hear a fire alarm while sitting in your office, which prompts you to get up and leave your office.

You hear the alarm because your ears detect the sound and relay signals to the brain's auditory center. Immediately, without your conscious awareness, your brain recognizes that this sound is a fire alarm because the sound of the alarm activates the memory of fire alarms past. Your brain then seeks to detect the smell or sight of smoke to evaluate if there is a real fire nearby and, if necessary, to stop or *inhibit* other activity that you were engaged in (writing an email, talking on the phone, etc.). Other memories may be activated at the same time—for example, the memory that this is a mundane drill that you were notified about the day before. At that point, more brain systems come into play to provide spatial information about how to get out of your office and to move outside into a safe space.

Communication among these distinct systems—sensory processing, memory, and action planning—then causes your brain, and subsequently your muscles, to initiate a motor response. If you smell smoke, you'll run out of the building as fast as you can. If you realize this is just a drill, you may answer a few emails or stop by a colleague's office to say hi before you slowly walk out of the building. If you had previously experienced trauma in a context that involved fire, your brain may generate emotional and physical reactions of fear and anxiety, increased heartbeat, flashback of trauma memory, and freezing or startle response. All of these behaviors and reactions to a single sound can be generated because brain systems can communicate with each other and coordinate their activity. So how does the brain do this?

Neurons Are Cellular Computers

Around a hundred years ago, it became clear that the brain is composed of billions of individual cells that are closely connected with one another. These cells, called *neurons*, make up the functional units of the brain, and the connections between them are called *synapses*. A set of synaptically connected neurons can form a *network*, the activity of which represents almost anything—a sensation, memory, emotion, or behavior. For example, individual neurons may represent different sound frequencies. When these neurons are activated in a particular way, they can then synaptically activate other downstream neurons—for example, those that represent the memory of a fire alarm.

But how does one brain network selectively activate another one? The memory of a fire alarm is rapidly activated by a very specific sensory input, but rarely in other circumstances. This is possible because each neuron in the

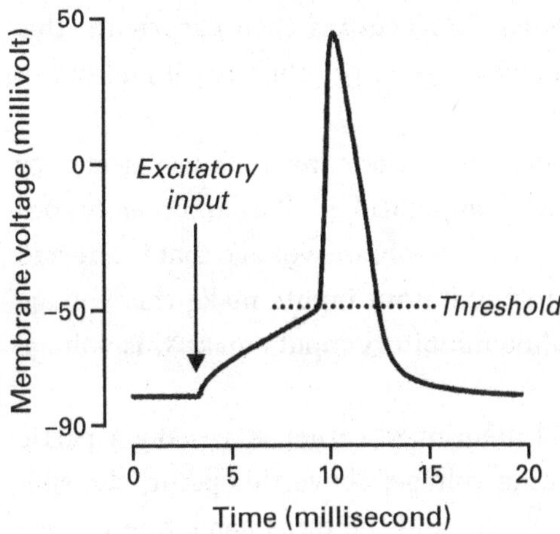

Figure 3 A neuron is excited or *fires* when the membrane voltage goes above a threshold. This is usually caused by another neuron providing an excitatory input via a synaptic contact.

brain acts as a *computer* that *integrates* signals from one or, much more commonly, many hundreds or thousands of other neurons. Neurons continuously monitor these inputs, which may be *excitatory* (proactivity) or *inhibitory* (prosilence). In some cases, if the neuron becomes excited to a certain *threshold*, it will *spike* and then send synaptic signals to downstream neurons (figure 3). Importantly, if a neuron does not spike, it generally does not signal to downstream neurons. This all-or-none spiking activity thus represents a *digital output*: it happens (1) or does not happen (0). Downstream neurons then experience this digital output as an excitatory or inhibitory input and respond in turn.

Also like modern computers, neurons use electricity as the basis for their computations.[1] The outer membranes of neurons have a transmembrane voltage that is affected by synaptic inputs: excitatory inputs make this voltage more positive, while inhibitory inputs make this voltage more negative.

The threshold mentioned earlier is actually a particular transmembrane voltage; above this point, the spiking machinery kicks in, and the transmembrane voltage rapidly (in less than a millisecond) becomes positive and then negative. The biophysics of the spike allow for the digital output of the neuron to be carried long distances as a self-propagating wave—for example, from one side of your brain to the other, or from your spinal cord to your pinky finger.

Neurons Communicate Using Neurotransmitters

To understand the mechanism of action of ketamine, we need to take a closer look at how brain cells signal to one another—that is, the process of *neurotransmission*. At synapses, the digital, all-or-none spiking output of one neuron (the *presynaptic* neuron) is transduced into the excitatory or inhibitory input felt by another neuron (the *postsynaptic* neuron). This occurs via a *chemical process*: when the presynaptic neuron spikes, it releases chemicals, called *neurotransmitters*, onto the postsynaptic cell (figure 4). Other types of neurons do not synapse onto other neurons; instead, they release neurotransmitters that can travel long distances in the brain and affect many cells simultaneously.

Neurotransmitters can be small molecules with few functions other than to facilitate communication between cells (figure 4). Examples of this class of neurotransmitters include dopamine and serotonin. But the majority of neurotransmitters are common amino acids, lipids, or small proteins called *peptides* that have a wide range of functions in the brain, as well as the rest of your body, in addition to acting as neurotransmitters. In the case of amino acids, for example, they are the building blocks of proteins.

Neurotransmitters Need Receptors to Communicate

After neurons release neurotransmitters, the neurotransmitter can only be recognized by the surrounding neurons if those neurons contain highly specialized proteins called *receptors*.[2] Therefore, it is not the neurotransmitter alone that is communicating with the surrounding neurons,

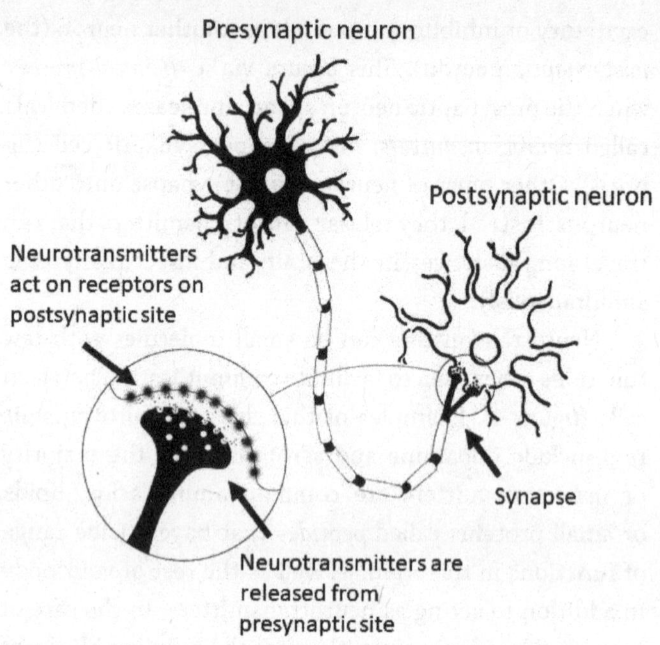

Figure 4 Neurotransmitter molecules are released from the presynaptic neuron when that neuron is excited. The neurotransmitter molecules then diffuse across the synapse to the postsynaptic neurons. There neurotransmitters facilitate communication with the postsynaptic neuron if they collide with receptors that recognize them. Neurotransmitters can be removed by a "reuptake" mechanism that involves transporter proteins moving them back inside the cell. They can also be metabolized by enzymes. Both of these processes reduce neurotransmitter numbers and therefore the probability that they will find and activate their receptors.

but the action of the neurotransmitter on a receptor. If a neuron does not have the receptor for a particular neurotransmitter, it is not affected by the release of that neurotransmitter. Importantly, however, receptors on neurons do not need natural neurotransmitters to be activated. A whole host of drugs (e.g., nicotine, opiates) that have similar structures to natural neurotransmitters can directly activate their particular brain receptors.

The brain is full of receptors for all kinds of chemicals: not just the neurotransmitters that are released rapidly at synapses and cause excitation or inhibition of surrounding neurons, but also hormones and other *modulatory* neurotransmitters that are released over time scales of seconds, minutes, and days.

The structures of receptors are highly specialized to recognize specific neurotransmitters (or drugs that have a similar chemical structure). A given neurotransmitter, such as serotonin, typically has multiple receptors that recognize it, but seldom do we have a brain receptor that recognizes more than one neurotransmitter. Depending on the receptor that is activated, a given neurotransmitter can have both rapid (excitatory or inhibitory) effects by acting on one subset of receptors and slow modulatory effects by acting on other types of receptors. Importantly, most receptors recognize neurotransmitters only when they are on the outside, but not on the inside, of the cell.

What happens when a receptor is activated? It depends. At a synapse, activation of fast excitatory receptors opens a path or a *channel* in which charged ions like sodium (Na^+) flow from the outside to the inside of the neuron. This flow of charged ions lasts for a few milliseconds, but that is enough to make the transmembrane voltage more positive and excite the cell, as shown in figure 3. This type of neurotransmission is optimized for fast, effective communication between neurons. By contrast, actions of modulatory neurotransmitter receptors occur over longer time scales: modulatory neurotransmitters and hormones generally do not directly cause excitation (or inhibition) of neurons. Instead, they generally initiate changes in signaling and gene expression that can cause long-lasting or even permanent changes in the neuron.

How Do Neurotransmitters Find and Activate Receptors?

The region of the receptor structure that is on the outside of the cell has specialized sections that neurotransmitters floating around in the extracellular space can recognize. The region that extends inside the cell also has specialized sections that define the downstream consequences of receptor activation.

Once they are released into the extracellular space, neurotransmitters find their receptors essentially by random collision (figure 4). When it finds the right receptor, a neurotransmitter can *fit* and briefly bind to the receptor. The probability that a neurotransmitter finds this region and binds to it increases with the increasing number of neurotransmitter molecules that are passing by the receptor: if there are several thousand versus a handful of neurotransmitter molecules that are passing by the receptor, the chances of a neurotransmitter molecule colliding with, and thus binding to, this site increases.

The binding of a neurotransmitter to the receptor can be very brief—a few milliseconds—or last up to tens of seconds. After that, the neurotransmitter detaches and moves on. This brief binding is sufficient to transiently change the structure of the receptor protein so that it becomes activated.

What determines the time course of neurotransmission? There are several key factors here. First, there is the tendency for neurotransmitters to diffuse in the brain's extracellular space after being released, just as food coloring diffuses throughout a glass of water. As time moves along, neurotransmitters become fewer and further between, less likely to activate a given receptor. Receptors close to the neurotransmitter release site are thus more likely to be activated than receptors distant from the release site. The brain can also terminate signaling by enzymatically breaking down neurotransmitters such that they do not activate their receptors or by reuptake pumps that literally pump the neurotransmitters back into the cell so they are unable to activate their surface receptors. Finally, some receptors become *inactivated* for a variety of reasons such that they cease to function even when bound to their neurotransmitters.

These factors, which are different for each neurotransmitter-receptor pair, enable a wide variety of signaling patterns that are critical for brain function. For example, a slow modulatory input might make a neuron more or less likely to spike for a given fast excitatory input, all other things being equal. These modulatory systems, which will be described in more detail here in the context of ketamine's effects, are important for brain processes like mood and motivation. For example, while fast-acting neurotransmission allows for sensations like sight and hearing, modulatory systems may trigger a period of vigilance or anxiety after experiencing a threat such as a fire alarm, promoting planning and decision-making long after the actual alarm has stopped.

Ketamine Acts on Many Brain Receptors

The principal actions of ketamine are assumed to be mediated by manipulating the function of a few brain receptors. It is important, however, to underscore that ketamine is considered a "dirty" drug, meaning that it can influence the function of a large number of proteins (and not just receptors) in the brain.

The list of brain receptors that ketamine can act on is long.[3] Ketamine influences the function of these receptors in two ways. First, it can mimic the function of a natural neurotransmitter that neurons release on some receptors. In this role, ketamine is an *agonist*: a man-made chemical mimicking the effect of a natural neurotransmitter. Second, ketamine can interfere with a neurotransmitter's ability to act on (or *bind* with) a receptor and thus block the effect of the natural neurotransmitter at that receptor. In this role, ketamine is an *antagonist*.

The *affinity* of ketamine for these brain receptors, meaning the concentration that is needed to activate a proportion of the receptors, varies greatly depending on the receptor type. Let's assume ketamine has high affinity for (hypothetical) receptor A and low affinity for (hypothetical) receptor B so that the same concentration of ketamine activates or blocks 95 percent of A receptors but 5 percent of B receptors. This, however, does not dictate that the action on the receptor with a higher affinity is causing key behavioral or clinical effects. If the brain function we are interested in is more dependent on receptor B than receptor A, then the small 5 percent effect on receptor B is actually more important for the biological effect.

Effects of Ketamine on Glutamate Receptors

Ketamine's highest-affinity interactions are with one of the receptors for the neurotransmitter glutamate.[4] Glutamate is a common amino acid (building block of proteins) and the most prevalent excitatory neurotransmitter in the brain. Nearly all networks in the brain rely on glutamate for synaptic transmission between neurons. As such, glutamate has been implicated in nearly all brain functions, ranging from simple reflex reaction to emotional regulation, memory consolidation, and complex cognitive constructs such as attention.

Glutamate is also heavily implicated in neurodegeneration and cell death. The overexcitation of neurons by glutamate, if gone unchecked, can damage neurons and eventually kill them. This phenomenon is called *excitotoxicity*. Because of this, the brain has reuptake pumps that rapidly, while using a lot of energy, transport released glutamate from the extracellular space back inside the cell to prevent it from stimulating too many receptors.

There are two major families of glutamate receptors, named for the synthetic chemicals (figure 5) that allowed for their discovery: *AMPA receptors* specifically bind a molecule called α-amino-3-hydroxy-5-methyl-4-isoxazolepropionic acid, while *NMDA receptors* specifically bind a molecule called n-methyl-d-aspartate (hence the abbreviation).[5] Both NMDA and AMPA receptors act

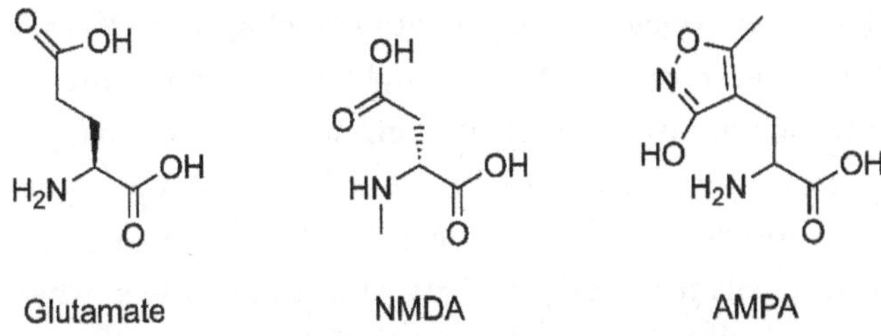

Figure 5 Synthetic chemicals that bind to receptors of glutamate. The respective receptors are accordingly called NMDA and AMPA.

as ion channels when they bind glutamate, allowing positively charged ions like sodium (Na^+) to flow into the cell. This causes a rapid change in membrane voltage, causing excitation of neurons.

AMPA and NMDA receptors differ in several respects. While AMPA receptors can always be activated by glutamate, NMDA receptors require at least two other events to be occurring in order for glutamate to bind and activate the receptor: (1) the neuron needs to be already excited by another receptor activation (e.g., by AMPA receptor activation), and (2) the amino acid glycine needs to be present at another site of the NMDA receptor. Thus, AMPA receptors form the basic "hardware" for excitatory synaptic transmission in neurons, while NMDA receptors are activated less frequently and only under specialized circumstances.

Moreover, NMDA receptors also allow for calcium (Ca^{2+}), an important signaling molecule, to enter the cell, which can trigger a host of other biological processes. NMDA receptors are thus thought to be important for learning because they trigger long-term cellular changes in response to coordinated neuronal activity. The regulatory constraints on NMDA receptor activation also help protect cells from excitotoxicity, which can happen when too much glutamate is released, NMDA receptors are overactivated, and toxic amounts of Ca^{2+} flow into the cell.

Among neurotransmitter receptors, ketamine has the highest affinity for the brain's NMDA receptor.[6] This means that for a given concentration of ketamine in the brain, NMDA receptors will be the most extensively bound by ketamine. At the NMDA receptor, ketamine is an *antagonist*, meaning that it blocks activation of the receptor.

How does ketamine block the NMDA receptor? Antagonists sometimes work by competing with the natural neurotransmitter for the binding site: they bind or occupy the space on the same site where the neurotransmitter binds but do not activate the receptor, thus preventing normal activation by neurotransmitter (figure 6). Ketamine, however, does not compete with glutamate but instead blocks the function of NMDA receptors in a very interesting way.

After glutamate has acted on the NMDA receptor and opened the channel, ketamine gets inside the receptor and blocks the channel itself, preventing the flow of ions like Na^{+} and Ca^{2+}. That means that in order for ketamine to act

Among neurotransmitter receptors, ketamine has the highest affinity for the brain's NMDA receptor.

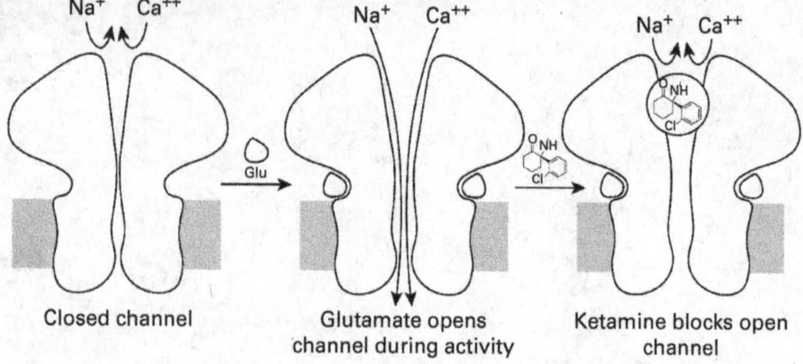

Figure 6 Simplified structure of the NMDA receptor. When glutamate stimulates the receptor, it opens a channel that allows positively charged calcium and sodium to move into the neurons and excite it. Ketamine blocks this effect by getting into the channel. Note that ketamine can only block the activity of NMDA receptors that are already stimulated by glutamate.

as an NMDA receptor antagonist, two sequential conditions have to be met.

First, the neuron that contains the NMDA receptor must have been excited by glutamate; second, glutamate must have subsequently bound to the NMDA receptor and opened the channel. It is only then that ketamine can go inside the channel and block it.

This unusual property makes ketamine a *use-dependent* receptor blocker. That essentially means that ketamine selectively blocks the function of neurons that are engaged in doing something but leaves the silent ones alone. This property may be key in how ketamine affects brain function.

Other drugs that activate or block brain receptors (including several other NMDA receptor antagonists) indiscriminately act on receptors regardless of the state of the neuron. But ketamine selectively targets networks of neurons that are engaged in specific functions. This could be an emotional or mood-related network that is producing reverberating thoughts, contributing to depressive symptoms or flashbacks related to PTSD.

Ketamine's Action on Glutamate Neurotransmission Can Cause Disinhibition of Neurons

Because NMDA receptor activation is excitatory and ketamine blocks this process, you would assume that the main effect of ketamine would be to silence the brain. However, this is not really the case as its effect depends strongly on the administered dose.

At high doses, ketamine is a powerful and rapid-acting anesthetic, consistent with a silencing action on brain activity. But at low doses, the opposite happens: ketamine *increases* neuronal activity. How? In several brain regions, NMDA receptors are present at high numbers on neurons that release inhibitory neurotransmitters. These neurotransmitters act on receptors that, similar to glutamate acting on AMPA receptors, open channels to allow charged ions to flow in the cell. The only difference is that instead of allowing in a positively charged ion such as Na^+, they allow negatively charged chloride (Cl^-) to flow into the neuron. This shifts the membrane voltage to the negative side and thus inhibits the neurons.

When glutamate activates the neurons that release inhibitory neurotransmitters, the downstream effect is inhibition of surrounding cells. This interplay of excitation and inhibition provides a balance that is important for information processing in the brain, especially for the so-called higher-order functions of cognitive and emotional processing and decision-making. By preferentially blocking the excitation of inhibitory neurons, ketamine indirectly increases overall neuronal activity: a process called *disinhibition*.

The first discovery that ketamine may in fact be having a disinhibitory effect came from the work of the author's lab where it was observed in laboratory rats that ketamine and similar drugs can increase glutamate and the firing rate of some neurons in the cerebral cortex.[7] This particular mechanism has been implicated in the antidepressant effect of ketamine, as will be discussed in chapter 4.

Effects of Ketamine on Other Brain Receptors

While much of the clinical effect of ketamine on depression or even its anesthetic effects are attributed to inhibition of the NMDA receptor, it is important to appreciate that as a dirty drug, ketamine can act on a wide variety of brain receptors. Even at low doses, ketamine's actions on these other receptor systems may cause some of its antidepressant effects, as these receptor systems are crucial for regulating motivation, mood, drug reward, and pain sensation.

One of these receptor systems recognizes *acetylcholine* as its natural neurotransmitter. Unlike glutamate, which is a ubiquitous amino acid, the function of the acetylcholine molecule is limited to its role as a neurotransmitter. At the *neuromuscular junction*, where motor neurons activate muscle contraction, acetylcholine is the primary excitatory neurotransmitter, analogous to glutamate's role in the brain. In the brain, however, acetylcholine neurons are not as prevalent as glutamate neurons, and the functions associated with acetylcholine are more specialized. These involve mostly higher-order brain functions such as memory, motivation, and attention.

Ketamine can act as an antagonist at multiple subtypes of acetylcholine receptors called *nicotinic* and *muscarinic receptors*. (The names come from the fact that these two receptor subtypes were first discovered after finding that natural compounds in tobacco, later found to be nicotine, and the hallucinogenic mushroom Amanita muscaria, later found to be muscarine, bind to them with high affinity.) The affinity of ketamine for the muscarinic receptors

As a dirty drug, ketamine can act on a wide variety of brain receptors.

is quite low but slightly higher for one of the subtypes of nicotinic receptor, called *alpha*-7.[8]

Other neurotransmitters with receptors targeted by ketamine are mostly ones that modulate the function of surrounding neurons. *Modulation* in this context means that stimulation of the receptor does not overtly excite or inhibit the receiving neuron. Instead, ongoing activity is tweaked. The implicated neurotransmitters in this context, whose receptors are influenced by ketamine, are dopamine, serotonin, and endogenous opiates.

Ketamine has low affinity at the receptors for the neurotransmitters serotonin and dopamine, which are important for the regulation of mood and motivation.[9] These interactions may include agonist properties at the serotonin 5HT2A receptor, which is the same receptor that is thought to be the site of action of hallucinogens LSD and psilocybin.

Ketamine has considerable affinity at several opioid receptors.[10] Opioid neurotransmitters are a group of peptides (small proteins) with multiple functions, including modulation of mood and sense of well-being and modulation of pain perception. Depending on the receptor subtype, ketamine has both agonist and antagonist properties. Ketamine's actions on these receptors likely contribute to its acute analgesic (pain-reduction) properties. Recent studies also suggest that the antidepressant effects of ketamine may be mediated by actions on opioid receptors.[11]

Finally, recent studies show that ketamine may also influence the function of a subtype of estrogen receptor called *ER-α* (ER alpha).[12] *Estrogen* is a hormone that is released primarily by the ovaries and is generally associated with female sexual maturation and reproduction. In the context of the ER-α receptor, it is important to underscore that ovaries are not the only source of estrogen. Neurons in both male and female mammalian brains can make estrogen and express receptors that are activated by it. The functions of these receptors are diverse and include regulation of release of multiple neurotransmitters, including dopamine and serotonin. While many of these effects are observed in both males and females, some of the effects, including activation of dopamine release, appear to be stronger in females.

Ketamine's affinity for estrogen receptors may be as potent as its affinity for the NMDA receptor. Thus, low doses of ketamine used for treating depression are likely to significantly influence the function of this receptor. Activation of hormone receptors often entails a longer duration of action (minutes to hours to days) compared to the rapid (millisecond to seconds) activation of NMDA receptors. A single bout of activation of hormone receptors can be sufficient to make changes in gene expression that last for days. An estrogen-mediated mechanism may therefore have relevance for any long-term impacts of ketamine (several days), including its antidepressive effects. Depression is far more prevalent in women compared to men, and the general consensus (though statistically adequate studies remain lacking) is that ketamine is more effective in treating depressive symptoms in women than men.

Modulating Neurotransmission through Mechanisms Other Than Receptors

In addition to acting on receptor proteins, ketamine modifies the action of proteins that can indirectly influence the function of neurons. For example, ketamine interferes with the proteins that transport neurotransmitters such as dopamine and serotonin out of the extracellular space.[13] This enhances the effects of these neurotransmitters because it lets them stay longer outside neurons and continue to stimulate their receptors. Ketamine also increases the release of dopamine for several hours after a single injection. Mechanisms for this effect are a matter of debate, but regardless, the released dopamine can then bind with dopamine receptors and further enhance dopamine-mediated neurotransmission.

Another indirect way that ketamine can influence neurotransmission is by stimulation of the activity of an enzyme called *acetylcholinesterase*. This enzyme metabolizes the neurotransmitter acetylcholine. Similar to glutamate, acetylcholine can be neurotoxic if it lingers for too long after it has been released. However, instead of energy-expensive pumps to move it out of the extracellular space (as is the case with glutamate), the brain uses an enzyme to metabolize and thus deactivate acetylcholine.

Acetylcholinesterase is one of the most powerful enzymes in all biological systems, with each enzyme molecule breaking down about a thousand acetylcholine molecules per second. (Of note, albeit unrelated to ketamine, many deadly nerve gases such as sarin work by inhibiting acetylcholinesterase, overloading the neuromuscular junction with acetylcholine and preventing muscle contraction.) The ability of ketamine to stimulate acetylcholinesterase is quite long lasting, reportedly persisting for several hours after a single dose. Activation of this enzyme promotes breakdown of acetylcholine, causing a reduction in neurotransmission mediated by all of its receptors. This effect may contribute to the cognitive and memory deficits and potential neurotoxicity that accompany use of ketamine.

While many of these non-NMDA effects are considered weak, there could be an additive effect. Thus, ketamine could be influencing brain function through a perfect storm of manipulating multiple neurotransmitter systems.

Ketamine and Non-neuronal Entities in the Brain

Neurons are not the only cells in the brain. There are a whole host of other cells that provide functional support to neurons. Chief among them are a class of cells called *glial cells* or *glia*. There are multiple types of glia, with both specialized and generalized functions. Some of these functions include supporting and insulating neurons and their branches, removing dead neurons, supplying oxygen and other nutrients to neurons, and delivering immune response–related chemicals needed to destroy pathogens.

In the context of glutamate neurotransmission and NMDA receptor–mediated functions, glia play a significant role in keeping glutamate levels in check.[14] Recall that cells can constrain neurotransmission by pumping neurotransmitters out of the extracellular space. The majority of energy-demanding pumps that remove glutamate from the extracellular space after it is released from surrounding neurons are located on glial cells. Efficient removal of glutamate is critical for shortening the duration of NMDA receptor activation, thereby also impacting the effectiveness of ketamine, which blocks the NMDA receptor in a use-dependent manner. The role of glia, however, may extend beyond clearing glutamate. There is a rapidly evolving literature that shows ketamine may influence the function of different subtypes of glial cells (astroglia and microglia) to influence a whole host of events that regulate how glia influence extracellular ion and glutamate homeostasis.[15]

Metabolites of Ketamine Can Influence Brain Function

Ketamine, like most drugs, is metabolized by liver enzymes. With ketamine, this metabolism is extensive, leading to numerous metabolic byproducts.[16] These metabolites are important in the context of the behavioral and therapeutic effects of ketamine for multiple reasons. First, some of them may contribute to the therapeutic effects of ketamine. For example, the metabolite norketamine exerts anesthetic effects that may allow for the maintenance of anesthesia after ketamine itself has been metabolized. Another metabolite, 6-hydroxynorketamine, has been shown to exert antidepressant effects in preclinical models.[17] This suggests that ketamine metabolites might work on brain systems independent from ketamine.

Second, some metabolites may lead to potentially dangerous or unexpected interactions when other drugs are taken together with ketamine. This often happens because the same liver enzymes are responsible for breaking down multiple drugs. Some of these enzymes are present in limited quantities, and if two or more drugs are competing for the same enzyme, less of each may be broken down. In this context, a known example is that combined administration of antianxiety drugs such as diazepam (Valium) or Xanax with ketamine slows down clearance of both drugs and exacerbates their sedative effects.

Third, there are *polymorphisms* (the presence of genetic variation within a population) in genes coding for some of the liver enzymes that break down ketamine. This means that there is interindividual variability in how well these drug-metabolizing enzymes work to break down ketamine. Depending on the dose of ketamine used, this can have clinically important consequences. Little is known about the impact of the genetic variation of these enzymes on the antidepressant effects of ketamine, but some recent studies have established a link between the genetic variation of one of these enzymes (CYP2B6*6 allele) and the rate of clearance of ketamine in chronic pain patients.[18]

Effects of Ketamine on Energy Metabolism

For reasons as yet unclear, repeated exposure to ketamine changes the levels of compounds involved in multiple energy and amino acid metabolic pathways. This has been best characterized in laboratory studies in rodents and macaque monkeys. These studies show that blood serum levels of multiple amino acids (leucine, threonine, alanine, glycine, etc.), fatty acids (propanoic acid, butanoic acid), cholesterol, and intermediate substrates in energy metabolism such as phosphates, pyruvate, lactate, and urea are affected.[19] While it is not clear how these changes may contribute to the desired clinical effects and potential side effects of ketamine, the large impact on metabolically relevant molecules should not be dismissed. Brain has a high energy demand and, more than any organ in the body, is sensitive to fluctuations in metabolism that may result in changes in the energetic status of cells.

Behavioral Effects of Single or Repeated Use of Ketamine in Laboratory Animals

Ketamine is used widely as a tool in neuroscience to probe the impact of NMDA receptor blockade on behavior. The published studies involve use of laboratory animals, as well as human volunteers.

Ketamine continues to be used as an effective and relatively safe veterinary anesthetic. But at subanesthetic doses, it has an interesting and stimulatory behavioral profile in laboratory animals. In rodents (rats and mice), subanesthetic doses produce increased locomotor activity and a distinct pattern of repetitive movements.[20] Animals (rodents and monkeys) learn to self-administer ketamine, confirming that it provokes pleasant sensations and may have abuse potential.[21]

Subanesthetic doses also produce cognitive deficits in laboratory animals that are quite similar to those reported in human subjects. These include deficits in attention, memory, and decision-making. Because of these similarities, ketamine and related drugs (especially PCP) have been used as animal models for some aspects of schizophrenia.[22]

The animal studies have helped delineate some of the mechanisms that may account for behavioral effects of ketamine in humans. The cognitive and memory effects are likely to be primarily mediated by inhibition of NMDA receptors. The indirect effects of ketamine on dopamine and serotonin, which are independent of its NMDA inhibitory effects, may play a role in the euphoria and motivation of animals to self-administer it.

There is a large body of peer-reviewed scientific research in laboratory animals on the impact of ketamine and similar drugs, especially PCP, after chronic and subchronic exposure. In these studies, *chronic* generally refers to frequent, often daily exposure for many weeks, and *subchronic* refers to daily exposure for several consecutive days or intermittent exposure for several weeks. Obviously, the exposure regimen in rats and mice is difficult to compare to human dosing. For example, rats and mice live for only two to three years, and their entire adolescent period lasts less than a month.[23] Thus, two weeks of daily exposure in rats may be equivalent to months of exposure in humans. Regardless, these studies are useful for understanding potential mechanisms that may be involved in any adverse effects of repeated exposure to ketamine.

The animal literature shows that some of the adverse effects of ketamine are exacerbated or *sensitized* over time.[24] This includes the erratic movement of rodents about their cage and worsening of cognitive deficits, including short- and long-term memory. On the other hand, repeated exposure to ketamine produces tolerance to anesthetic and pain-reducing effects of ketamine, suggesting that higher doses or more frequent dosing may be necessary to reach the desired effect.[25]

Potential mechanisms for these adverse behavioral (including cognitive) effects are diverse. Multiple mechanisms—including disruption to the brain immune response, changes to specific neurons and neurotransmitter systems in the brain, increases in astrocytes (a type of glial cell), and lasting changes in the function of proteins key in regulating glutamate neurotransmission—have been implicated.

Behavioral Effects of Single or Repeated Use of Ketamine in Humans

At subanesthetic doses, ketamine generally causes a state of mild intoxication, characterized by a sense of dissociation from the environment and alterations of speech, hearing, and vision. These doses can be associated with anxiety, as well as dream-like imagery that contributes to its euphoric effect in some individuals. The same doses are also associated with cognitive deficits influencing attention, memory, and decision-making.[26]

Physical signs of low-dose intoxication include muscular discoordination and disorientation. The combined cognitive deficits, dissociation, and psychosis-like effects such as hallucination have been the rationale to use these low doses as a model of schizophrenia in clinical laboratories. Importantly, these effects are often perceived as pleasant, and ketamine at these doses remains a popular drug for recreational use.

At higher doses, but still subanesthetic, the motor effects are exacerbated, causing great difficulty in moving and some respiratory disturbances. These doses can produce more profound dissociation from reality, loss of consciousness, and intense hallucinations. This state has been referred to as a near-death experience or the K-hole. Seizures and nausea can be associated with these doses.

At anesthetic doses, ketamine's effect is short lasting.[27] While emerging from ketamine anesthesia, ketamine can cause an intense reaction characterized by hallucinations and delirium. This is often called an *emergence state* and is characterized by a sense of confusion, dissociation from reality, and changes in perception. Ketamine can also causes transient memory impairment.

Studies on the impact of long-term use of ketamine are rare. Clinical use of ketamine as an anesthetic or in human laboratories as model of schizophrenia typically involves a single dose of ketamine. Because of this, our knowledge of the impact of repeated use of ketamine is either from animal studies or from individuals who repeatedly use ketamine recreationally. The latter data are somewhat unreliable because ketamine is often abused in combination with other drugs, such as cocaine, methamphetamine, alcohol, and benzodiazepines like Valium. It is therefore difficult to delineate the effects of ketamine as all these other drugs have profound effects on brain function. Regardless, some of these studies indicate that repeated exposure to ketamine may lead to sustained psychiatric symptoms, including anxiety, hallucinations, paranoia, disorganized thought, and emotional withdrawal, which can persist for several days following use.[28] Nonpsychiatric symptoms associated with repeated use involve renal function and urinary track pathologies such as ulcerative cystitis. Mechanisms for these effects are not well understood but may be due to some of the metabolites of ketamine.

A few studies have reported on populations of pure ketamine abusers. These studies, albeit limited, indicate that repeated ketamine use may cause lasting changes in dopamine receptors in the cerebral cortex and changes in brain connectivity in association with mild cognitive and memory impairment.[29]

4

KETAMINE AS AN ANTIDEPRESSANT

About Depression

Major depressive disorder (MDD) encompasses a group of debilitating brain illnesses, including major depression. The term *major depressive disorder* was introduced by American clinicians in the 1970s and became part of the official clinical diagnostic terminology in *DSM-III* in 1981.[1] DSM is an acronym for *Diagnostic and Statistical Manual of Mental Disorders*. The current edition is *DSM-5* and remains the primary tool for diagnosis of depression and other mental illnesses.

In North America, MDD has a staggering lifetime prevalence that by some accounts exceeds 14 percent of the population. The incidence may be on the rise, especially in adolescents and the elderly. This is a disconcerting trend: MDD, in addition to affecting personal, social, and professional functioning, can be deadly because it is strongly associated with increased incidence of suicide.

Symptoms of depression are complex and extend beyond feelings of sadness or unhappiness. These symptoms must last at least two weeks for a diagnosis of depression. Symptoms include but are not limited to the following:

Loss of interest or of feeling pleasure in activities that were once enjoyable

Changes in sleep, appetite, weight, and energy level

Irritability and agitation

Difficulty in concentrating and making decisions

Feelings of worthlessness or guilt

Changes in motor function that range from an increase in purposeless movement (pacing) to a decrease in purposeful acts (slower speech and walking)

Thoughts of death and suicide

Depression is not a new malady. The term *melancholy* has been used to describe the same devastating illness for centuries.[2] What is new is the alarming trend in increased rates of suicide that are associated with depression. According to the US Centers for Disease Control and Prevention (CDC), rates of suicide in the US have increased by 33

Depression is not a new malady. The term *melancholy* has been used to describe the same devastating illness for centuries.

percent in the last ten years. It is currently the second leading cause of death for adolescents to thirty-four-year-olds.

Symptoms of depression in some individuals are alleviated effectively with nondrug approaches, including psychotherapy and cognitive behavioral therapy.[3] Other noninvasive interventions, such as lifestyle changes, including increasing physical activity and mindful meditation, have also been shown to be effective in subsets of patients.[4] But as the focus of this book is on ketamine, we will focus on drug and other invasive treatments for MDD.

Current Standard Drug Treatments for Depression

Multiple classes of antidepressant medications such as Prozac are used currently to treat general depression and other MDD. But while some patients respond effectively to them, about 30 percent do not.[5] All these antidepressant drugs are the same or analogs of drugs discovered accidently in the 1940s and 1950s (discussed in more detail ahead). They can take up to several weeks of daily dosing to start producing their antidepressant effects. How they work to reduce symptoms of depression and why prolonged treatment is needed to reach their clinical efficacy remain to be understood.

The history of how the current antidepressant drugs were discovered and gained popularity for widespread

Multiple classes of antidepressant medications such as Prozac are used currently to treat depression. But while some patients respond effectively to them, about 30 percent do not.

clinical use is an interesting combination of serendipitous discovery of drug effects by scientists, and clinicians with a shrewd instinct for marketing within the pharmaceutical industry. This business model has persisted for decades and was applied again for marketing esketamine as a new antidepressant. The reliance of scientists and pharmaceutical companies on animal models developed to explain the effect of these accidentally discovered drugs, as opposed to understanding the biology of the illness, has contributed to few, if any, of the current medications used to treat psychiatric disorders being truly novel.

History of Treating Depression

The condition of *melancholy* had been used in medical textbooks for centuries to describe patients who were a fixture of asylums, with symptoms similar to major or psychotic depression. The first drug to be used for treatment of depression is most likely opium: there is recorded use of poppy seeds to enhance mood as early as the second millennium BC. Avicenna (Ibn Sina), an Iranian physician-philosopher, mentioned its use in his medical encyclopedia, *The Canon of Medicine*, which was completed in 1025 and used through the eighteenth century in Europe.[6] The practice continued through the Victorian age and modern-day Europe as laudanum became readily available without

Reliance on accidentally discovered drugs, as opposed to understanding the biology of the illness, has contributed to few of the current medications used to treat psychiatric disorders being novel.

prescription. Laudanum, a tincture of opium developed in the sixteenth century that includes the naturally occurring alkaloids morphine and codeine, remains available in the United States by prescription.[7]

The profound addictive properties of opiates clearly did not make them a sustainable approach to treat depression. But then came the introduction of electric shock therapy, later named electroconvulsive therapy (ECT), in the 1940s. This treatment offered an intervention for severely depressed patients for the first time. One application of ECT could immediately relieve the intense feelings of sadness and hopelessness in these patients for weeks. Despite the side effect of varying degrees of memory loss, ECT became a staple for treatment of severely depressed patients in the 1950s.[8]

As a side note, ECT treatment is not as dramatic (or cruel) as the name implies. Popular media and the portrayal of the procedure dramatized in books and movies such as *One Flew Over the Cuckoo's Nest* have contributed to the perception that this is a barbaric and cruel procedure. Modern-day application of ECT involves providing patients, who have given consent to the procedure, general anesthesia and muscle relaxers before the procedure. Calibrated electrical current is then applied over the skull via pads.[9] ECT provides immediate relief in symptoms of severe depression in patients who have not responded to other modes of therapy.

How ECT works to rapidly alleviate symptoms of depression remains an enigma. Recall that neurons communicate by getting excited or inhibited due to shifts in voltage across their membrane. ECT, therefore, could be changing the excitability of neurons in the areas of stimulation. But how does this cause relief of symptoms of depression? Multiple theories have been proposed and continue to be refined as our knowledge of fundamental neuroscience increases.[10] These remain theories, however, and no studies to date have shown a clear mechanistic relationship between passing a jolt of current through the skull and immediate alleviation of depressive symptoms.

Use of ECT in the 1950s happened against the backdrop of increased clinical use of newly discovered psychoactive drugs. These included the first modern antipsychotic, chlorpromazine (Thorazine), for patients with schizophrenia.[11] It also included an attempt by the pharmaceutical industry to find new uses for newly discovered compounds. One of these included Benzedrine, an amphetamine initially marketed by Smith, Kline & French (SKF) as a decongestant. Benzedrine became popular as a mood and energy enhancer, initiating the so-called pep pill industry—in part, because SKF marketed the drug to family physicians as a treatment for mild depression. As the use of Benzedrine soared, SKF developed another amphetamine, Dexedrine, a structural analogue of Benzedrine, to offset the impact of Benzedrine going off patent. But while use of these amphetamines in individuals diagnosed by family physicians as having mild depression was prevalent, there was little evidence that they helped alleviate symptoms of major depression.

At the same time, and on the other spectrum of drug effects, another class of drugs with sedative or tranquilizing effects became popular. These drugs were dubbed *minor tranquilizers* and were used to treat *neurosis*, later called *anxiety*. First in this class of drugs was meprobamate (with two brand names: Miltown, developed by Carter-Wallace Pharmaceutical; and Equanil, developed by Wyatt). Soon after meprobamate was introduced to the market, it became the bestselling drug in the history of the United States.[12] Informally called the *peace pill* and *emotional aspirin*, Miltown was liberally prescribed to and consumed by 1950s professionals and became synonymous with the emergence of self-medication in the so-called cold war age of anxiety. (This area became even more successful in the 1960s with development and marketing of Valium by Hoffmann-La Roche.)

First Marketed Fast-Acting Antidepressant Drug

While tranquilizers such as Miltown did not improve depressive symptoms, the fact that many patients with depression suffer from anxiety offered a new marketing opportunity for pharmaceutical companies: a mixture of amphetamines, to enhance mood and energy, and barbiturates, to take the edge off the agitation and anxiety.

These mixtures were marketed as "rapid" and "prompt" treatment for depression (figures 7 and 8). The company that seized this opportunity first was SKF. In 1950, SKF began to market Dexamyl, a mix of amylobarbitone (a barbiturate sedative) and Dexedrine (an amphetamine). Magazine ads of the era marketed Dexamyl "for proved antidepressant effects—both rapid and prolonged." Next came Deprol, developed by Wallace Pharmaceuticals, the maker of Miltown. Deprol was a mix of Miltown and benactyzine also heavily marketed for treating "symptoms of depression and associated anxiety." Deprol became widely used by family physicians for rapid-acting "treatment of endogenous depression."

Use of these drugs for treatment of chronic depression did not persist for multiple reasons. First, they were not generally effective. While some drug-company-sponsored trials suggested they were effective, subsequent trials did not find amphetamines effective for treating symptoms of depression. Second, their safety came into question, with incidents of mortality being reported.[13] Finally, novel classes of drugs began to emerge that, while slow acting, demonstrated better clinical efficacy in treating symptoms of depression.

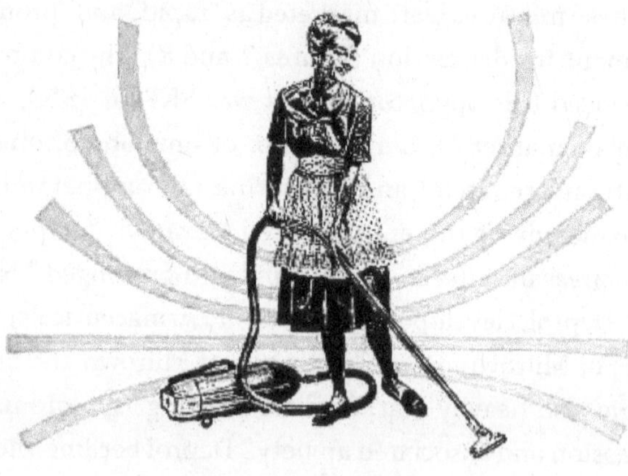
for proved antidepressant effect—
both rapid and prolonged
DEXAMYL® SPANSULE®
brand of dextro amphetamine and amobarbital
brand of sustained release capsules
'Dexamyl' has been used successfully for over a decade, and in sustained release form for more than six years. Just one 'Dexamyl' *Spansule* capsule, taken in the morning, provides daylong therapeutic effect. And mood elevation is usually apparent within 30 to 60 minutes.
'Dexamyl' is of significant value in depressed and verbally inhibited patients. Drayton[1] states, "Not only does ['Dexamyl'] exert a direct mood effect, so that the shadow of depression is lifted, but it also results in making the patient more approachable and communicative."
1. Drayton, W., Jr.: Pennsylvania M. J.
leaders in
psychopharmaceutical research

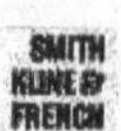
SMITH
KLINE &
FRENCH

Figure 7 Drug company advertisement for rapid-acting antidepressant actions of Dexamyl, with mood elevation apparent within thirty to sixty minutes. Dexamyl was marketed by Smith, Kline & French starting in 1950. It was a mixture of a barbiturate sedative (amylobarbitone) and an amphetamine (Dexedrine).

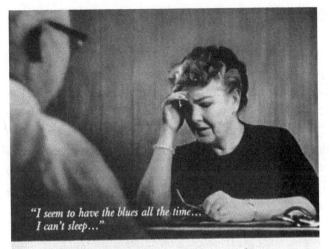

in the depressed, unhappy patient

PROMPTLY IMPROVES MOOD

without excitation

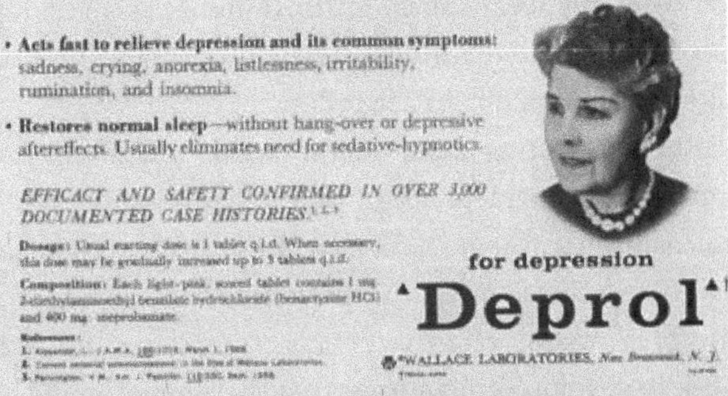

Figure 8 Advertisement for Deprol, indicating that "it acts fast to relieve depression." Deprol, developed by Wallace Pharmaceuticals, was a mix of Miltown, a popular sedative and antianxiety mediation, and benactyzine, a stimulant.

Emergence of Present-Day Antidepressant Drugs

In the early 1950s, reports that the antituberculosis drug iproniazid (marketed under names Marsilid and Rivivol) had profound euphoric and mood-enhancing properties in TB patients prompted psychiatrist Nathan Kline to use this drug to enhance the "psychic energy" of patients with depression. The initial clinical trials reported positive results, prompting the FDA to approve Marsilid as the very first drug to specifically treat "symptoms of endogenous depression."

After the FDA approval, Marsilid was prominently used as an antidepressant drug. It was, however, withdrawn from the market a few years later because of serious hepatic toxicity side effects.[14] About the same time, another drug, developed by the Swiss-based pharmaceutical company Geigy as an antihistamine, was accidently discovered to have antidepressant properties. That drug, imipramine, remains in use today.

The interesting story of the accidental discovery of imipramine's antidepressant properties is as follows. The clinical observation in 1952 that the drug chlorpromazine has antipsychotic effects in patients with schizophrenia prompted many pharmaceutical companies, including Geigy, to develop similar drugs that they hoped would have antipsychotic properties. Chemists in Geigy, a few years earlier, had synthesized imipramine as an antihistamine, but its structural similarities with chlorpromazine promoted them to test the drug in patients with schizophrenia. This relatively large-scale study involving several hundred patients, led by Swiss psychiatrist Ronald Kuhn, failed to show that imipramine has a significant effect in improving psychosis. But Kuhn noticed an improvement in a few patients who also suffered from depressive symptoms, prompting him to test the drug in a subsequent clinical trial with patients with severe depression. The results, reported in 1957 and published in 1958, were impressively positive—particularly because, in contrast to the transient jolt of euphoria produced by stimulants, imipramine produced lasting and normalizing effects on mood and behavior.[15]

After this discovery, Geigy quickly began to market imipramine under the trade name Tofranin.[16] This followed an approval in 1959 by the FDA for treatment of depressive and other mood disorders. Soon, other pharmaceutical companies followed suit with similar drugs. Tofranil remains in use as one of the *tricyclic antidepressants*, so named because the chemical structure of this class of drugs includes three fused carbon rings.

The mechanism of action of tricyclics remains unclear to this day. They act on multiple sites in the brain, including receptors for the neurotransmitters noradrenaline, serotonin, dopamine, acetylcholine, and histamine. More recently, they have been dubbed serotonin-norepinephrine reuptake inhibitors, or SNRIs. The newer SNRIs, such as duloxetine (trade name Cymbalta), have a similar mechanism of action as these older drugs. Tricyclics remain some of the most efficacious of antidepressant drugs but generally are not well tolerated. They cause sedation and have multiple unpleasant side effects, including dry mouth, blurred vision, and constipation. They may also prove to be deadly because of the cardiotoxicity associated with an overdose.

Although Marsilid was withdrawn for use as an antidepressant because of its hepatic side effects as tricyclics entered the market, it remains in use to treat TB. Laboratory-based studies with this compound showed that in the brain, it blocks the activity of the enzyme, monoamine oxidase (MAO). This enzyme metabolizes the so-called monoamine neurotransmitters (serotonin, dopamine, and noradrenaline) after they are released by neurons, thus shortening their duration of action. This discovery led to the first neuro-centric hypothesis about depression. The so-called monoamine hypothesis of depression posited that low levels of circulating monoamines are associated with depression.[17] Inhibition of the MAO alleviated symptoms of depression by reducing the metabolism of monoamines and thus increasing their availability to stimulate their receptors. Based on this, it was proposed that depression results from reduced resting levels of monoamine neurotransmitters. Subsequently, tricyclic antidepressants were found to influence the function of monoamine neurotransmitters. Interestingly, amphetamines, the fast-acting antidepressant of the 1950s, and ketamine, the fast-acting antidepressant of the current era, both have MAO inhibition properties (albeit with low affinity).

Some MAO inhibitors remain on the market as antidepressants, but while they are not as dangerous as Marsilid, they have serious side effects, including causing hypertensive crisis and psychosis in some patients. They also have dependence-producing effects, causing withdrawal symptoms if use is discontinued abruptly.

Prozac Enters the Market

Despite the serendipitous discovery of MAO inhibitors and tricyclic antidepressants, the next generation of antidepressants entered the market somewhat by design. Basic research into the mechanism of existing antidepressants in the 1960s was beginning to suggest that increasing serotonin neurotransmission may be a unifying pathway for the clinical effects of these drugs. Serotonin is a prevalent neurotransmitter in the brain that influences many functions, including mood and sleep.

This effort was primarily led by Arvid Carlsson, at the University of Gothenburg in Sweden, who made the discovery that effectiveness of the existing antidepressants correlated best with their ability to block the pump that transported serotonin back to the neuron. As reviewed in chapter 2, when neurotransmitters are released by neurons, the brain often has mechanisms for clearing them rapidly to regulate the timing of their ability to stimulate receptors. This regulation is critical for optimal brain function because if the neurotransmitter hangs around too long, it can lead to excessive stimulation of receptors. On the other hand, if neurotransmitters are removed too fast, their function will be suboptimal.

For monoamine neurotransmitters, such as serotonin, clearance mechanisms are primarily governed by two mechanisms. One is by enzymes, such as MAO, that degrade and thus inactivate the neurotransmitter molecule. The second is by their transporter proteins, which literally pump the neurotransmitter molecule out of the extracellular space.

The discovery by Carlsson led to the development by Astra pharmaceutical in 1971 of zimelidine (trade name Zelmid), the first selective serotonin reuptake inhibitor (SSRI) for treating depression. The rationale for developing SSRIs was that by selectively increasing serotonin neurotransmission, one could achieve clinical efficacy while avoiding side effects. This was a logical design because most enzymes, including MAO, have many neurotransmitter substrates, so their effect is not necessarily neurotransmitter specific. Transporters, on the other hand, are generally quite specific for a given neurotransmitter.[18] Thus, blocking the transporter protein provided a mechanism whereby serotonin neurotransmission could be selectively enhanced without affecting the function of other neurotransmitters.

Zelmid showed excellent clinical efficacy in treating depression but was withdrawn from the market in 1983 because it was found to be associated with the potentially fatal Guillain-Barré syndrome. By then other pharmaceutical companies, in particular Eli Lilly and Company, were developing and testing similar compounds.[19] The first of these drugs to clear research and development (R&D) and get approved by the FDA for treatment of depression was fluoxetine (trade name Prozac) in 1987.

Prozac became a sensation and highly profitable for Eli Lilly. In 2001 alone, it generated three billion dollars in sales. This success led other drug companies to develop and introduce to the market equally popular SSRIs (e.g., Zoloft, Paxil, and Celexa). Despite the popularity of Prozac and other SSRIs, it is critical to underscore that their clinical efficacy to treat symptoms of depression was not better than the older drugs. What made them popular was that they have fewer side effects than the tricyclics and MAO inhibitors and therefore are better tolerated.[20]

Little Progress Is Made after the Introduction of Prozac

While Prozac and other existing antidepressant drugs have made a tremendous difference in the lives of many who suffer from depression, about 30 percent of patients do not respond to the current medications or cannot tolerate the side effects. This has led to continued efforts in the last fifty years to develop better drugs that target novel sites in the brain.

Efforts to discover more efficacious antidepressants have included intense laboratory-based academic research supported by the National Institutes of Health (NIH) and private foundations, along with resources allocated to R&D by major pharmaceutical companies. But the new SSRIs and SNRIs currently on the market use the same mechanisms as the older drugs developed decades ago. The antidepressant drug development field essentially remained stagnant after the introduction of SSRIs until the reports of the antidepressant effects of ketamine.

Why did fifty years of research fail to develop novel targets for depression? There are multiple guesses. One is that models used to study depression in basic research contexts are not adequate. The animal models (mostly mice and rats) used to assess depressive-like symptoms often involve arbitrary approaches of inducing a state of helplessness and aversion. Classic tests included housing rodents with aggressive cage mates, prolonged swim

The antidepressant drug development field essentially remained stagnant after the introduction of SSRIs until the reports of the antidepressant effects of ketamine.

sessions (rodents can swim, but they don't like it), or repeated exposure to various stressful contexts. While these paradigms are relevant to a general state of distress, clinical signs of depression are far broader than feeling stressed or unhappy about your environment.

Another limitation has been that theories that led to emphasis on SSRI, SNRI, and MAO inhibitors created a simplistic view of the neuroscience of depression. Specifically, as mentioned earlier, because all existing antidepressants increase levels of serotonin and/or noradrenaline (by reducing their uptake into cells in the case of SSRIs and SNRIs or by reducing their metabolism in the case of MAO inhibitors), the prevalent theory became that there is reduced monoamine (in particular, serotonin and noradrenaline) neurotransmission during depression that is corrected by these drugs. While there may be some validity to this simple model, there were several inconsistencies with this model. The most glaring one is that these drugs increase serotonin levels robustly a few minutes after a single dose, whereas the antidepressant effects often do not take effect until several weeks of repeated treatment.

Another key inconsistency with the serotonin or monoamine model of depression relates to the results of clinical studies that experimentally reduced serotonin production in patients with depression and control subjects. How was this done? The method to reduce serotonin neurotransmission in humans was pioneered at the Yale

Department of Psychiatry in the late 1980s, with some of the key papers emerging in the early 1990s.[21] The design was straightforward. Serotonin is synthesized from the amino acid tryptophan. Tryptophan is one of the handful of *essential* amino acids, meaning that the body cannot synthesize it, so it has to be provided through diet. A carefully controlled diet devoid of tryptophan for as short as twenty-four hours reduces brain serotonin production.

The studies at Yale were led by Pedro Delgado, who was a psychiatry resident at the time under the intellectual leadership of two giants in biological psychiatry, George Aghajanian and George Heninger, also known as the Two Georges. Aghajanian had performed some of the fundamental basic science work related to this approach as the first person to record from serotonin, noradrenaline, and dopamine neurons of mammals; and Heninger directed the psychiatry clinical unit that was pioneering translational approaches to treating mental health. Another psychiatrist researcher involved in these studies was Dennis Charney, who played a role later in ketamine trials for depression.

The gist of the findings of the initial tryptophan-depletion studies, supported subsequently by more elaborate studies, was that transiently depleting brain serotonin does not cause depression in healthy subjects.[22] This questioned the idea that reduced serotonin neurotransmission alone is responsible for causing depression. But the researchers did find that serotonin depletion worsened symptoms of some patients with depression. This worsening did not occur during the tryptophan depletion, however, when serotonin synthesis and release would be low. It usually occurred with a delay and after return to normal tryptophan in diet, and only in a subset of patients. This indicated that serotonin levels did not have an immediate or causative relationship with depression and that any effect is related to neuronal events downstream from serotonin release.

Serotonin and Monoamine Models of Depression Persevere

The emerging literature questioning a causative relationship between reduced serotonin and depression led to modified theories. These theories, however, remained serotonin-centric and did not lead to discovery of novel targets. Specifically, the field focused on downstream and delayed effects of antidepressant drugs. For example, these newer theories posited that an increase in serotonin neurotransmission by antidepressants causes various forms of neuroplasticity, or lasting changes, in other downstream pathways that then produce antidepressant effects.

One of these theories capitalized on findings by Robert Sapolsky at Stanford and the late Bruce McEwen at Rockefeller that chronic stress in lab animals, which some researchers use as a model of depression, can reduce the arbor-like processes on neurons that are used to make contact with surrounding neurons.[23] This phenomenon is guided by reduced secretion of a so-called growth factor, the brain-derived neurotrophic factor (BDNF), and could be reversed if BDNF was injected directly into the brain.[24]

Growth factors such as BDNF are proteins or steroid hormones that, as the name implies, are involved in cellular growth, proliferation, and repair. BDNF is one of the more prevalent and best-characterized growth factors in the brain and plays a role in both neurodevelopment and survival of neurons after development. Similar to neurotransmitters, growth factors work primarily by acting on membrane-bound receptors. BDNF works through a receptor called TrkB. These receptors are localized on neurons throughout the brain and play a key role in multiple functions, including neuronal survival.

The discovery that BDNF plays a role in the detrimental effects of chronic stress on neuronal processes generated interest in the depression field and led to hypotheses that this factor may be involved in depression and the clinical efficacy of antidepressant drugs.[25] The subsequent finding that SSRIs increase BDNF levels in laboratory animals further supported this hypothesis.[26]

While the hypothesis that antidepressant drugs work through changing BDNF levels remains mainstream, postmortem data from patients with MDD is not generally supportive of BDNF levels being low.[27] Some studies have shown that BDNF is not disrupted at all, whereas some show disrupted BDNF levels in multiple brain disorders in addition to MDD, including schizophrenia, dementia, and bipolar disorder. The strength of postmortem studies is often limited because of low subject numbers and other confounds such as a history of drug use. But a recent study with a large number of subjects showed that lower BDNF levels was selective to those patients with MDD that also suffered from dementia. No differences were seen from control subjects in the MDD group without dementia.[28]

The BDNF and other newer theories of depression continued to have the same shortcoming as monoamine theories, in that they were driven by the logic that how antidepressants treat symptoms reveals what is causing depression. Often in medicine, the relationship between symptom alleviation and disease etiology are unrelated. For example, while opiates may alleviate the pain symptoms of tooth decay, the decay is caused by an infection, not insufficient stimulation of opiate receptors. Years of research effort expended on understanding the pain-reducing effects of opioid drugs and opiate receptors would not enhance our understanding of the etiology and physiology of dental cavities. Similarly, years of focusing on how antidepressants work has not put us any closer to understanding the causes of depression.

Discovery of the Antidepressant Effects of Ketamine

There had been anecdotal reports of ketamine enhancing mood since its use as an anesthetic during the Vietnam War, but the first clinical trial of ketamine to treat depression was not published until 2000. This was a limited study (only seven subjects) conducted at the West Haven VA Medical Center by Yale-affiliated scientists. The study's researchers reported in a peer-reviewed journal that a single dose of ketamine can have a rapid onset effect in ameliorating some symptoms of depression.

Concurrent with this study, ketamine was being used as a research tool by John Krystal and colleagues at the West Haven VA Medical Center and Yale to model some aspects of schizophrenia. This approach was based on findings many years earlier that the ketamine analog phencyclidine (PCP) produces schizophrenia-like symptoms in healthy individuals. At the time of these early findings, we knew little about how low doses of PCP and ketamine, which were developed as anesthetics, affect behaviors that are relevant to schizophrenia. The later discovery that subanesthetic doses of PCP (and ketamine) block the NMDA receptor revolutionized the mechanistic thinking about

There had been anecdotal reports of ketamine enhancing mood since its use as an anesthetic during the Vietnam War.

schizophrenia in that it suggested that schizophrenia may involve a disruption in the function of the NMDA receptor or, more generally, glutamate neurotransmission in some brain regions.

This mechanism remains viable because recent genetics and imaging data collected from patients with schizophrenia suggest a malfunction of some glutamate receptors. Indirect verification that a reduction in glutamate function at the NMDA receptor causes psychosis and some of the symptoms of schizophrenia is supported by the condition called NMDA-receptor encephalitis (beautifully described by Susannah Cahalan in the book *Brain on Fire*).[29] This autoimmune disease essentially destroys NMDA receptors in the brain. The symptoms of the early stages in which NMDA receptors have been partially inactivated have an uncanny resemblance to schizophrenia. Many patients suffering from this illness are initially diagnosed with schizophrenia until the symptoms of the advanced stages of the illness, in which overt seizures (caused by near-complete lack of functional NMDA receptors) not typically seen in schizophrenia begin to emerge.

The purpose of using low-dose ketamine as an experimental model of schizophrenia was to gain an understanding of possible brain pathways that may be dysfunctional in schizophrenia (chapter 2). This was the primary motivator for Krystal to begin to characterize behavioral effects of ketamine in healthy volunteers. These individuals were administered subanesthetic doses of ketamine as their behavioral response was monitored. It was found that ketamine transiently disrupted behavior in a manner that mimicked some symptoms of schizophrenia.[30] Follow-up visits with the subjects that received a ketamine treatment suggested no long-term adverse effects, with some reporting a positive impact on mood.

In addition to a focus on schizophrenia, the West Haven VA Medical Center-Yale group at the time had a strong emphasis on studying major depression and other mood disorders. After the 2000 study, however, antidepressant effects of ketamine were not studied further until six years later by a group at the intramural program at the National Institute of Mental Health (NIMH). Lack of follow-up by the Yale group could have been in part because, at the time, ketamine studies in humans were facing negative press, implying that overzealous researchers were intentionally making people sick by giving them ketamine. In addition, well-controlled double-blind clinical trials with sufficient subjects to produce meaningful results are expensive, often putting them out of the reach of single academic institutions.

At the time of the first ketamine studies by Krystal, his boss (the chief of psychiatry at the West Haven VA Medical Center) was Dennis Charney, who a few years later moved to NIH as the scientific director of NIMH. Charney's research interests primarily involved MDD. While at Yale, he had been involved in the tryptophan-depletion clinical studies, as well as the first limited ketamine trial. Access to the resources of the intramural program allowed Charney and his new team to begin to refocus on ketamine's antidepressant effects. The work, now led by Carlos Zarate and Husseini Manji at the NIMH intramural program, reported the first randomized, placebo-controlled, double-blind study with ketamine in treatment-resistant patients in 2006, showing a rapid antidepressant effect resulting from a single intravenous injection of ketamine.[31]

Making Ketamine Profitable

In 2006, Charney (who had since left NIMH to become the dean of research at Mount Sinai School of Medicine), Krystal, Manji, and Zarate filed a patent for intranasal administration of ketamine for treatment of depression (application S78510806P filed by Yale University, NIH, and Mount Sinai School of Medicine). Ketamine had been used off-label for years, but the nasal spray method of administration could offer a path to a patent, thereby making an old drug profitable. Manji soon moved to Johnson & Johnson as the head of global therapeutics in neuroscience at Janssen Research & Development. Janssen, a subsidiary of Johnson & Johnson, spearheaded the efforts to get FDA approval for ketamine for treatment of depression.

Making ketamine profitable was not trivial. Its use patent expired years ago and generic versions commonly used as an anesthetic are available for literally a few dollars.

Ketamine is an old drug. Its use patent expired years ago, and many generic versions commonly used as an anesthetic are available for literally a few dollars. A fifty-milliliter bottle of one hundred milligram/milliliter concentration of ketamine, which should be enough for over fifty injections of the antidepressant dose of ketamine, is generally less than fifty dollars. Key to making ketamine lucrative was to use the nasal spray preparation *and* to shift from ketamine to one of its stereoisomers S-ketamine (esketamine). As discussed in chapter 1, ketamine is what is called a *chiral compound*: it is a mix of two molecules, or two isomers, that are mirror images of each other. These molecules have the same atoms and general structure but, like left and right hands, are not superimposable. The left- and right-handed versions of ketamine are called R-ketamine (arketamine) and S-ketamine. In general, unless (R)- or (S)- is specified, the word *ketamine* refers to what is called a *racemic mixture* containing equal parts (R)- and (S)-ketamine.

Esketamine had been shown to have a higher affinity as an NMDA antagonist and is a more potent anesthetic and psychosis-inducing compound. Interestingly though, animal studies have provided some evidence suggesting that arketamine may be a better antidepressant and less toxic.[32] Supporting this idea, the only human study to date that compared the effect of S- and R-ketamine in healthy individuals reported that while esketamine produced

Key to making ketamine lucrative was to use the nasal spray preparation *and* to shift from ketamine to one of its stereoisomers esketamine.

psychosis-like symptoms and delirium, arketamine produces a state of elation and euphoria, suggesting that it would be a more effective isomer for producing antidepressant effects.[33]

The decision by Johnson & Johnson to proceed with patenting the S isomer, therefore, does not seem to have been guided by published clinical data. It is possible that this was due to the difficulties of patenting arketamine or simply because esketamine was easier to manufacture. It may also have been assumed that a higher affinity for blocking the NMDA receptor would result in better antidepressant properties.

The first clinical trial in depression with esketamine was carried out by Johnson & Johnson/Janssen investigators and financially supported entirely by that company. The study was published in the journal *Biological Psychiatry* (editor in chief, John Krystal) in 2016. Johnson & Johnson marketed the intranasal esketamine under the name Spravato and began efforts for FDA approval.

The FDA approved use of Spravato for treating depression in March 2019. At the time of approval, only three relatively small studies with ketamine had been completed. One of these studies had shown a significant effect in alleviating symptoms of depression. The other two did not. This topic will be discussed in greater detail in chapter 6.

Since the initial published reports of the antidepressant effects of ketamine, multiple investigators at many universities and government-associated hospitals, as well as in the pharmaceutical industry, have been conducting clinical trials with ketamine or esketamine for treating depression and suicide ideation. There are currently nearly three hundred ongoing or completed registered clinical trials related to ketamine and depression. Many of these studies are now completed. The gist of the findings generally can be summarized as follows: in a subgroup of treatment-resistant patients, ketamine and esketamine decrease symptoms of depression for a few days.

HOW DOES KETAMINE PRODUCE ANTIDEPRESSANT EFFECTS?

NMDA Receptor Is the Star of the Show

Reports of fast-acting effects of ketamine on treatment-resistant patients quickly stimulated neuroscience research seeking a novel mechanism to explain its antidepressant effects. Many theories have proliferated, thanks in part to ketamine's "dirty" mechanism of action involving a large number of receptors.

Older antidepressants act primarily on proteins that influence the function of neuromodulators such as serotonin and noradrenaline. For example, SSRIs such as Prozac block the function of the protein that moves serotonin back into the cell after it is released. Ketamine is being touted as different because it could be acting on an entirely different neurotransmitter system (glutamate) and protein (NMDA receptors) to produce its antidepressant properties. Accordingly, a large number of laboratory-based studies have proposed new models to explain how ketamine's actions on the NMDA receptor could cause antidepressant effects.

At lower subanesthetic doses, which are the doses typically used to treat depression, ketamine is assumed to act primarily on one of the most prominent receptors in the brain, the NMDA receptor. As reviewed in chapter 3, NMDA receptors are one of the subclasses of receptors activated by the excitatory neurotransmitter glutamate. Ketamine blocks the function of this receptor in an activity-dependent manner, meaning that the receptor first needs to be activated by glutamate before ketamine can block it.

Ketamine does not exclusively act on the NMDA receptor. There are a whole host of other receptors in the brain (chapter 3) that can be stimulated or inhibited by ketamine. But because these effects may be weaker at subanesthetic doses of ketamine, most of the theories and experimental approaches to study the antidepressant effects of ketamine have revolved around its action on the NMDA receptor.

Using state-of-the-art methodologies and mechanistic approaches, neuroscientists have shown that a single dose of ketamine can influence neuronal activity of specific brain regions, alter multiple intracellular signaling systems, and even modify brain morphology. But because

Older antidepressants act primarily on proteins that influence the function of serotonin and noradrenaline. Ketamine could be acting on an entirely different neurotransmitter system.

of the ubiquitous presence of NMDA receptors throughout the brain, the fact that ketamine or other NMDA antagonists can exert this multitude of effects is not surprising. The challenge has been how to isolate any of these ketamine-induced changes as relevant to antidepressant properties of ketamine.

To address this, laboratories have relied on the effects of ketamine in rodent models that may be relevant to depression. Of course, rodent models have serious limitations in the context of studying depression, which may be a uniquely human illness. But these models rely on two plausible and logical approaches that are related to human depression. The first approach capitalizes on the knowledge that repeated exposure to stress, especially unpredictable stress, often exacerbates and may even cause depression. The second takes advantage of rodent behavioral models that were used successfully decades ago to identify and screen classical antidepressants such as Prozac.

Animal stress models use experimental manipulations that involve repeatedly stressing the animals, such as exposing them to social isolation. A related approach mimics the hormonal effects of stress (instead of manually imposing stress) by injecting them with sustained high levels of the hormone corticosterone. This is the rodent version of the human cortisol that is secreted during stress exposure, among other conditions. The impact of these manipulations is then assessed on various measures of brain function. These could include recording neuronal activity in various brain regions, changes in receptor function or other proteins that are involved in signal transduction in neurons, and morphology of specific subtypes of neurons in regions of the brain suspected to play a role in depression. Then the impact of a single dose of ketamine is measured on these changes. The idea is that if ketamine reverses any of these effects, then that effect is relevant to antidepressant properties of ketamine.

The second approach is to use the so-called rodent behavioral models of depression. This has been a controversial approach because of the implications that they actually model depression. But these models have been quite prevalent in the field of antidepressant research because they were developed to successfully screen older drugs, including SSRIs. These behavioral models generally involve placing rats or mice in an aversive situation where escape may seem possible to them. The animal's continued mobility is measured as a sign of struggle to escape ("normal" behavior) versus giving up ("depressive" behavior), with the assumption that a lack of motivation to struggle or to escape resembles symptoms of depression. These tests include the forced swim test or tail suspension test.

Using these general approaches, several NMDA-centric theories about ketamine's antidepressive effects have been proposed. These involve data-supported mechanisms that we will call *theories* because, while they provide interesting facts about the effects of ketamine in rodents, direct data linking these mechanisms to the rapid but transient antidepressive effects of ketamine in humans is lacking.

One of the first theories proposed was by the Yale group who also initiated the clinical studies of ketamine.[1] Previously, the effects of ketamine had been attributed to its ability to actually *increase* glutamate neurotransmission despite blocking the NMDA glutamate receptor. This was based on data showing that ketamine and PCP could *increase* extracellular levels of glutamate and preferentially *inhibit the firing rate of inhibitory neurons*. It was then proposed that blocking NMDA receptors preferentially reduced the activity of inhibitory neurons, reducing inhibition of surrounding neurons. This phenomenon is also called *disinhibition*. Reduced inhibitory activity causes excitation and activity of other neurons, some of which can release glutamate and subsequently increase glutamate neurotransmission, especially through non-NMDA receptors such as the AMPA receptor.[2]

The Yale group, led by the late Ron Duman and George Aghajanian, proposed that this mechanism is also responsible for the antidepressant effects of ketamine. By increasing AMPA receptor–mediated neurotransmission, they proposed that ketamine (indirectly) increases BDNF levels, similar to classical antidepressants.[3] A key experiment to support this mechanism tested that chronic stress reduces BDNF levels, which they hypothesized contributes to symptoms of depression. Of note, this mechanism was similar to that used by the same group to explain the antidepressant activity of classic antidepressants such as Prozac. The supposed burst of glutamate release and AMPA receptor activation caused by NMDA-antagonist-induced disinhibition then restored the depleted BDNF level. One of the consequences attributed to restoring BDNF levels was that neuronal atrophy caused by chronic stress could be reversed.

A similar theory was proposed with ketamine using chronic cortisol injection as a model of depression. Specifically, injecting mice repeatedly with corticosterone causes atrophy of neuronal processes and reduces BDNF levels in correlation with effects on escape behavior. Ketamine treatment reversed these detrimental effects of corticosterone.[4]

This proposed mechanism has many strengths. First, because it involves ketamine's direct effect on the NMDA receptors, these receptors need to be activated before ketamine can block them (chapter 2). This will dictate that ketamine will selectively target active circuits of the brain and leave the silent ones alone. This is important because nonspecific actions on all NMDA receptors throughout the brain could be associated with unwanted side effects and generalized reduction on brain activity. This is also consistent with mechanisms described by Sapolsky, McEwen, and others decades ago that showed chronic stress can have detrimental effects on neuronal processes via the NMDA receptors. Thus, the fact that an NMDA receptor antagonist blocks this neuronal atrophy is not surprising and has been seen in multiple contexts.

One potential inconsistency, however, is that stress itself causes profound glutamate release, much more so than ketamine.[5] If the potential disinhibition-induced glutamate release by ketamine was an initial step to cause the antidepressant effect, then stress should have antidepressant properties. That is clearly not the case. Another inconsistency, discussed ahead, is that so far clinical trials with other NMDA receptor antagonists as antidepressants have failed.

An entirely different mechanism related to ketamine and NMDA receptors was proposed by Lisa Monteggia in 2011.[6] Her group reported that ketamine can act on the NMDA receptor independent of its action as an open channel blocker. As discussed in chapter 2, NMDA receptors contain an ion channel that opens when glutamate binds the receptor on an actively firing neuron. Ketamine blocks the NMDA receptor by getting inside an active and open channel. But the mechanism proposed by Monteggia does not depend on ketamine getting inside an open channel and could involve the NMDA receptor at rest. The functional consequence of this action was initiation of a cascade of intracellular events that involve deactivation of an enzyme called eukaryotic elongation factor 2 kinase (eEF2K). Deactivation of this enzyme then results in other downstream effects that also include increased expression of BDNF. This mechanism therefore was similar to the one proposed by Duman and Aghajanian in that a downstream effect involved BDNF, but the means to get there were different. The implication of the Monteggia model is that the effects of ketamine are not dependent on the NMDA receptor per se, and any other mechanism that can deactivate eEF2K, regardless of the receptor used, should have antidepressant properties.

Another NMDA-independent mechanism involves actions of one of the major metabolites of ketamine, hydroxynorketamine (HNK). In mice, HNK produced similar but longer-lasting effects on cellular and behavioral "antidepressant" measures compared to ketamine.[7] A cleaner NMDA antagonist did not have similar effects to ketamine, suggesting that mechanisms other than NMDA receptor blockade are responsible for the antidepressant effects of ketamine. The effects of HNK are, however, blocked by AMPA receptor blockade, suggesting that ketamine acts by increasing glutamate release and AMPA receptor–mediated neurotransmission. Interestingly, HNK also acts on eEF2K, suggesting the same downstream intracellular mechanisms are involved regardless of the initial mechanism.

Other related mechanisms involve more specific sites of action of ketamine. These *circuit-based* approaches assume that ketamine's action as an antidepressant depends on preferentially influencing NMDA receptor functions in select brain regions that are involved in regulating mood and motivation. These approaches usually take advantage of human postmortem or brain imaging data showing that the function of specific brain regions may have been compromised in patients with depression.[8] Scientists then specifically look for changes in those brain areas using animal models that can allow them to dig into potential mechanisms. For example, human imaging and postmortem studies have implicated a tiny region deep down in the brain called the habenula in depression.[9] These have been followed by studies in mice showing that ketamine can specifically influence the impact of stress in this brain region.[10]

Inconsistencies with Proposed NMDA Mechanisms of Action of Ketamine

Despite the wealth of the laboratory-based findings, recent data from clinical trials are questioning the basic assumption that NMDA receptors or related changes in glutamate neurotransmission are responsible for the antidepressant properties of ketamine.

Rodent models propose ketamine works as an antidepressant by acting on the brain's NMDA receptor. But so far, other drugs acting on NMDA receptors have not produced antidepressant effects.

The most convincing way of testing the idea that ketamine treats depression by blocking NMDA receptors is to compare its effect in a clinical trial with other drugs that also block the NMDA receptor. Several studies have done exactly that, and none have found that NMDA antagonists other than ketamine can treat depression. One study, in fact, compared ketamine with five other drugs that had NMDA-receptor-blocking properties; of these, only ketamine showed antidepressant effects.[11]

Some of the NMDA antagonist drugs used in these studies were older compounds with low selectivity for the NMDA receptor. A recent high-profile large-scale study, supported by the drug company Allergan, tested a new drug called rapastinel with selective affinity for the NMDA receptor as an antagonist. Animal studies had suggested that rapastinel has a very similar profile as ketamine.[12] This trial also convincingly failed to produce antidepressant properties in patients.

Other trials that assessed downstream systems that might be affected by the NMDA antagonist properties of ketamine have also been negative. Specifically, several laboratories had proposed that it may not be the NMDA receptor inhibition per se that causes the antidepressant properties, but downstream effects following NMDA blockade, such as secondary activation of the glutamate receptor AMPA or downstream signal transduction molecular mechanisms related to changes in BDNF (chapter 3).

But so far, clinical trials with drugs that target those sites have failed as well. A major recent trial with the experimental drug ORG26576, an AMPA receptor potentiator, failed to produce clinical efficacy in patients with depression. Another experimental drug, TAK653, with a similar mechanism to ORG26576, is currently under testing—but after over one year, results have been slow to come out. Finally, a drug that targets the molecular downstream effects of ketamine (BDNF-mTOR) called rapamycin also failed in a small trial to mimic the effects of ketamine in treating depression.[13] It is important to point out that both AMPA receptor signaling and mTOR signaling are widespread throughout many cell types and networks in the brain, so it is difficult to make clear biological interpretations of these studies.

Collectively, the negative results of multiple clinical trials with drugs that laboratory research predicted should work are disappointing and not consistent with the theory that NMDA receptor blockade by ketamine is the key mechanism for its antidepressant effects.

Other Potential Models to Explain the Antidepressant Effect of Ketamine

Given the negative outcome of the clinical trials discussed earlier, it is critical to underscore the fact that ketamine has an affinity for a large number of proteins other than the NMDA receptor in the brain. It may therefore be producing its antidepressant effects on treatment-resistant depression through entirely different mechanisms than those described earlier. Some of these mechanisms are listed ahead.

Neuroinflammatory Mechanisms

The anesthesia literature has long shown that ketamine may have anti-inflammatory properties. Ketamine reduces the production of some pro-inflammatory compounds including the so-called cytokines.[14] In the context of depression and MDD, this property is not trivial because immune-related mechanisms have been implicated in the causes and effects of depression. For example, elevated levels of peripheral inflammatory markers such as cytokine interleukin-6 (IL-6) or C-reactive protein (CRP) have been reported consistently in patients with depression. Moreover, positive response to traditional antidepressant drugs, such as SSRIs, reduces this elevation, suggesting that these drugs may owe some of their therapeutic effect to their anti-inflammatory properties. Along the same lines, elevation of these inflammatory markers is most prevalent in treatment-resistant depression.

Clinical data on the impact of ketamine on inflammatory markers in patients with treatment-resistant depression have recently begun to emerge. The number of these studies is limited, but so far they support a positive correlation between improvements in depressive symptoms and changes in cytokine levels after ketamine infusion.[15] Parallel animal studies are suggesting multiple NMDA-receptor-dependent and -independent mechanisms to explain the impact of ketamine on brain inflammatory mechanisms.[16] These studies usually implicate a role for glial cells in the brain, which provide support and immunological defense to neurons, in ketamine's effects in animal models of depression.

Estrogen Receptor

The biological role of estrogen is not limited to its effect as an ovarian hormone. Estrogen is produced in the brain by neurons, which have the machinery to convert cholesterol to estrogen. This includes neurons in the hippocampus, a brain region implicated in the pathophysiology of depression and the therapeutic impact of antidepressants. Similar to other neuromodulators, estrogen produces its effects in the brain by stimulating selective receptors. The common one in the brain is called *estrogen receptor alpha* (ERα), which is expressed in both male and female brains. ERα receptors are what are called *transcription factors*, meaning that their stimulation can directly produce lasting effects on gene expression. Optimal stimulation of these receptors has been linked to memory, mood, neuroprotection, and neurotoxicity.

Ketamine is a strong activator of ERα.[17] In fact, ketamine's affinity to stimulate ERα may be higher than its affinity for blocking the NMDA receptor. Importantly, inhibition of NMDA receptors is generally short lasting (minutes), thus making the lasting effects of a single-dose effect of ketamine on symptoms of depression difficult to reconcile. In contrast, stimulation of ERα receptors, by virtue of their being transcription factors, could have impact for days or weeks on gene expression and thus on brain function.

Opiates

The fact that opioids improve mood and can very rapidly alleviate symptoms of depression is well established. The recorded medical practice of treating melancholia with opium dates back to the late 800s. Developing opioid drugs that alleviate depression without producing their well-known detrimental addictive properties continued through the 1980s. Some of the current US opioid crisis may be attributed to the powerful effect of this class of compounds to elevate mood and rapidly produce a state of well-being.

As reviewed in chapter 2, ketamine acts on multiple opioid receptors. The affinity of esketamine for these opioid receptors is much higher (two- to fourfold higher) than arketamine. This has led some scientists to investigate a possible role for opioid systems in the antidepressant effects of ketamine. Interestingly, the effect of ketamine on animal models of depression (discussed earlier) does not appear to be mediated by opioids. Recent clinical studies, however, provide a different outcome. Specifically, treating treatment-resistant depressed patients with the opiate receptor antagonists naltrexone and naloxone (aka Narcan, ReVia or Vivitrol, used to counteract opioid intoxication) blocked the antidepressant and antisuicidal effects of ketamine.[18] Naltrexone did not block the dissociative and other effects of ketamine, suggesting that opioids may selectively mediate the antidepressive effects of ketamine.

ECT-Like Effects

A single dose of ketamine and ketamine-like drugs produces transient excitation of neurons and glutamate release in the cerebral cortex. This was first shown in laboratory animals. Human studies measuring cortical activity with functional MRI confirmed this transient excitation of cortical activity. This effect may mimic what happens during electroconvulsive therapy (ECT), in which currents are directly applied to the skull over select areas of the cerebral cortex. Similar to ketamine, ECT produces a rapid onset of antidepressant effects on treatment-resistant patients that last for days to weeks. In fact, a recent randomized controlled clinical trial comparing the therapeutic efficacy

Ketamine acts on multiple opioid receptors, and its antidepressant effects can be blocked by naltrexone.

of ECT and ketamine showed nearly identical therapeutic effects with both treatments.[19] The impact of ECT was longer lasting, but ketamine had the advantage of not causing lasting memory loss as sometimes occurs with ECT. While the mechanisms of the antidepressant effects of ECT remain elusive, this head-to-head comparison indicates that ketamine may be rapidly alleviating symptoms of depression via similar mechanisms.

6

SAFETY CONCERNS WITH KETAMINE AND ESKETAMINE

FDA Approval of Esketamine

The relatively speedy approval of esketamine (Spravato) by the FDA for treatment of depression raised a number of concerns. First among these was that the clinical efficacy of the drug was weak. In fact, the final ruling document released by the FDA after the approval stated, "There does not appear to be a consistent statistically significant positive primary efficacy outcome for Spravato-treated patients compared to placebo-treated patients." Translated, this means that even in the eyes of the FDA, Spravato was not consistently more effective than placebo.

The second concern—discussed ahead—was a lack of sufficient safety data about esketamine, especially in long-term use.

The vote on the FDA advisory committee that recommended the drug for approval was not unanimous. Two out of the sixteen members of the committee voted against approval, and one of the board members, Kim Witczak, took the unusual step of writing an editorial criticizing the rush to approval by the FDA.

In approving Spravato as an antidepressant drug, the FDA ignored the usual practice of requiring at least two successful placebo-controlled clinical trials. At the time of approval, Spravato had been tested in only four small trials and showed significant efficacy compared to a placebo in only one short-term trial. The FDA accepted the one successful trial and added on another trial with limited subjects and potentially flawed design. The data that have emerged subsequently with Spravato have not been any more impressive. In addition, while some individuals purportedly had a profoundly positive therapeutic result with ketamine, the overall therapeutic effect of esketamine in the few positive trials is relatively weak compared to placebo.[1]

What justified this quick approval path by the FDA? Spravato was marketed by Janssen pharmaceutical company, a subsidiary of Johnson & Johnson. The strategy it applied to speed up the approval process was to use the disease label *treatment-resistant depression* (TRD) instead of major depressive disorder (MDD). This allowed them

In approving Spravato as an antidepressant drug, the FDA ignored the usual practice of requiring at least two successful placebo-controlled clinical trials.

to obtain the FDA's fast tracking or breakthrough therapy designation. The FDA's fast-track route to approval was initiated in 1997 to make experimental treatments for serious and often terminal illnesses available more efficiently. This route is often used to approve new experimental therapies for advanced stages of cancer when other treatments have failed. This accelerated route essentially allows drug companies to make drugs available to patients without the same degree of rigorous testing in normal approval pathways.

TRD is responsible for substantial morbidity and mortality, including increased rates of suicide, which has been used to justify TRD as a potentially terminal illness and target for breakthrough therapy. The impact of esketamine on suicide prevention, however, was not convincing at the time of the approval. In fact, according to FDA advisory committee member Kim Witczak, there were cases of suicides that occurred during the clinical trials, but these were ignored and presented as unrelated to ketamine.

To this day, convincing data that esketamine prevents or reduces suicide risk are lacking. While several small studies with ketamine suggest it may help with suicide prevention, so far this does not seem to generalize to esketamine. A recent comprehensive randomized trial of Spravato in nearly four hundred patients at imminent risk for suicide showed no significant treatment difference with the placebo group. Even with ketamine, after several years of clinical trials in patients with depression, there is little data to convincingly establish that it reduces or prevents rates of suicide.

Cost

Ketamine solutions are cheap, around one to five dollars for a dose of racemic ketamine typically used to treat MDD. Initial studies reporting antidepressant effects with ketamine used a single dose, producing up to a week of antidepressant effects.[2]

The cost and recommended dosing for Spravato is a different story entirely. One dose of Spravato is currently $590 to $885, with three doses per week recommended to sustain the effect. (Johnson & Johnson has been projected to profit over $200 million from Spravato sales in the next three years.) In addition to the cost of the actual drug, there is the added cost of in-office administration, which includes two hours of monitoring for side effects including dissociation, hallucinations, and blood-pressure increases following administration. The treatment office must therefore employ multiple medical professionals equipped to handle hallucinatory, cardiac, and respiratory problems. The use of esketamine therapy may, therefore, incur substantial health-care-related expenditures even beyond the cost of the drug itself.

Esketamine and the VA

After the FDA approval of Spravato on March 5, 2019, it was quickly recommended for use in veterans within the US Department of Veterans Affairs (VA) healthcare system. The VA, which serves a large number of patients with TRD, could be an ideal proving ground for Spravato and a potentially lucrative market for Johnson & Johnson. The VA secretary at the time, Robert Wilkie, personally announced on March 19 that the VA will be making nasal spray available to veterans with depression. But that effort was stopped by a VA-affiliated panel of psychiatrists and researchers, who voted to not add Spravato to the VA's formulary (list of VA-approved medication) and to limit its use to preapproved, case-by-case treatment. The reason for their decision was not only that the overall effect of the drug was weak, but that there was no evidence from trials that it is effective in people over sixty-five, or even in males. Over half of VA patients are over sixty-five, and about 90 percent are male. There is also no safety data in this older population, raising the concern that esketamine is being rushed to use in veterans without proper evaluation of its safety.

The concerns of the VA board about the potential harm of continued use of a psychotropic drug with abuse potential, when there is a lack of safety data for long-term use, are not trivial. Regardless, President Trump ordered the

VA to order lots of ketamine, a move that raised eyebrows given the relationship of Johnson & Johnson executives with his campaign. The company had spent over $6 million in 2018 to 2019 to lobby the VA and federal government and contributed considerately to Trump's 2016 campaign. Despite the pressure from Mr. Trump, the restriction for use of Spravato in VA patients has been maintained as there remain serious concerns about the weakness of the evidence for clinical efficacy and lack of cost-benefit data.

Ketamine and Esketamine Have Unknown Long-Term Consequences

The recommended dosing for esketamine as an antidepressant is two to three times weekly for an indefinite duration.[3] Repeated dosing is recommended for more effective amelioration of suicidal ideation.[4] Thus, while the onset of antidepressant effects of ketamine and esketamine are reported to be fast, the effect wears off in a few days, necessitating continuous treatment.

Most of what we know about the neuroscience of ketamine is based on a single exposure of ketamine. Safety data for ketamine or esketamine use over a long period of intermittent exposure is lacking.

But should we be worried about the safety of repeated ketamine or esketamine use? After all, ketamine has been in clinical use as an anesthetic since the 1960s. The short-lasting psychosis-like effects notwithstanding, ketamine is generally assumed to be a "safe" drug. It is, however, important to keep in mind that all other clinical uses of ketamine, and therefore the ensuing safety assessments, have involved procedures that involve a single dose of ketamine.

The initial FDA approval of ketamine was for its sole use as an anesthetic. Anesthesia is typically a one-time treatment. Safety assessments of anesthetic drugs are generally limited to determining the lethal dose and potential side effects after exposure to a single dose of the drug. Thus, the initial FDA approval of ketamine did not include any safety information about its effect after repeated use. The clinical off-label use of ketamine (i.e., its use for purposes other than the FDA-approved use as an anesthetic) prior to antidepressant use also involved single or infrequent dosing. This involved use of ketamine to model psychosis in healthy volunteers or for pain relief. We know virtually nothing about the long-term consequences of indefinite two to three times per week dosing of ketamine or esketamine in humans.

Studies with ketamine in laboratory animals provide some disconcerting data about repeated use. These data are clearly limited for a variety of reasons, one being that lab studies mostly use mice and rats, which have much shorter lives than humans. How well does the two to three times per week dosing in animals model the use in humans for two to three months? These limitations notwithstanding, subchronic exposure (usually meaning once a day for three to five days) to subanesthetic doses of ketamine in rodents reveal long-lasting adverse effects, including neurotoxicity.[5] At the behavioral level, frequent administration of ketamine to rodents has been associated with cognitive deficits that include impaired short- and long-term memory.

The adverse effects of repeated ketamine appear to be worse in adolescents compared to adults in rodents and monkeys.[6] In addition, ketamine may impair normal development of the juvenile brain at both cellular levels and behavioral levels, including social behavior and memory.[7]

At this point, we have no idea how these laboratory studies will translate to humans and, unfortunately, are not likely to find out soon. While some published human studies include reports of adverse reactions to ketamine, none of these studies have offered cognitive or other behavioral assessments of individuals who received ketamine for days or weeks after the treatment has ended.

Fast to Act, or Quick to Relapse?

Traditional antidepressants start to produce their clinical effects slowly, typically after two to three weeks of treatment. Ketamine was lauded for being "fast acting" because, in some individuals, it produced its antidepressant effects within a few hours after a single dose. The emphasis on a single dose, however, is somewhat misleading because it implies that all you need to treat depression is that one dose. Most of the studies so far show, however, that patients relapse after a few days of receiving ketamine, necessitating another dose.

The rapid relapse and the need to continually administer ketamine or esketamine to maintain an antidepressant effect are hardly mentioned in media stories or press releases about the drug. Even animal studies that are now investigating the antidepressant effects of ketamine focus on giving animals one single dose and looking for permanent changes, as if assuming that the single dose was sufficient to cure depression.

When it comes to the time course of the antidepressant effect of ketamine (or esketamine), a fundamental problem may be that we are comparing it to other antidepressants, which generally take several weeks to take effect. We should, however, compare it to medications used to relieve physical pain, including opiates, steroids, or nonsteroidal anti-inflammatory drugs (NSAIDs). These drugs can rapidly alleviate pain, just like ketamine can alleviate symptoms of depression in some patients. But the effects wear off soon, necessitating repeated dosing. If we have learned anything from the so-called opiate crisis, it

The rapid relapse and the need to continually administer ketamine or esketamine to maintain an antidepressant effect are hardly mentioned in media stories.

is that the magical hype that these drugs are not addictive for treating pain was unfounded. While steroids and NSAIDs are not as dangerous, they also have been associated with profound long-term adverse effects that often emerge days and weeks after intermittent but repeated use has subsided. Is ketamine on the same trajectory?

Psychiatric and Cognitive Adverse Effects

Acutely, ketamine is associated with psychiatric disturbances, including hallucinations and delusions. While little data is available on the effects of repeated use of esketamine, the limited clinical data suggest that the psychiatric side effects are more intense and longer lasting with esketamine compared to arketamine or ketamine. These effects may worsen with repeated use, but they are not generally considered dangerous because they dissipate a few minutes or hours after use.[8] Studies in repeated ketamine abusers, however, have shown sustained impairment of short- and long-term memory.[9]

Genitourinary Tract Toxicity

A serious consequence of repeated ketamine (and esketamine) use may involve bladder disturbances and other abdominal, hepatic, and urogenital side effects. Data to support this come primarily from populations that use ketamine repeatedly for recreational purposes. While misuse of ketamine in North America and Europe pales in comparison to alcohol and opioids, ketamine has been a common drug of abuse in Southeast Asian countries, including China and Malaysia. In Hong Kong, ketamine was reported to be the most common drug of abuse in the early 2000s. Data from these populations have documented genitourinary tract toxicity in a considerable proportion of illicit ketamine users.

A condition commonly reported after repeated use of ketamine is ulcerative cystitis.[10] Symptoms of this condition involve painful hematuria (blood in urine), urinary urgency, and urge incontinence. This condition may require lifelong treatment, involving frequent cystoscopies and bladder catheterizations. It is unclear if such a condition is reversible after discontinued use of ketamine; surgical intervention may be required to maintain renal function.

Other side effects of repeated exposure to ketamine include hepatic and biliary abnormalities, along with a reduction in sperm motility.

Tolerance and Sensitization

The biological and behavioral effects of most psychoactive drugs change after repeated use. These changes can involve *tolerance*, referring to an effect decreasing with repeated use, or *sensitization*, referring to an effect increasing with repeated use. The same drug can exhibit both tolerance and sensitization on different effects.

In animal studies, ketamine and related drugs such as phencyclidine (PCP) produce both tolerance and sensitization. Repeated exposure to low subanesthetic doses of ketamine, PCP, and similar drugs causes what is called *locomotor sensitization* in rodents.[11] This refers to a gradual increase in spontaneous and purposeless movement, including running around the cage, rearing, and sniffing. This behavior is thought to be predictive of psychosis-inducing properties of these drugs because it can be blocked by antipsychotic drugs. In the context of repeated use of ketamine for treating depression, this potential effect may exacerbate and lengthen hallucinations and other dissociative side effects of ketamine.

Tolerance has also been reported for ketamine, but in that case, the targeted effect is the therapeutic anesthetic properties of ketamine. Specifically, after exposure to repeated dosing of ketamine over extended periods of time, higher and higher doses of ketamine are required to produce anesthesia or analgesia. Ketamine causes *self-induction* of multiple cytochrome P450 enzyme isoforms in the rat liver, increasing their ability to break down ketamine in the bloodstream. This suggests a mechanism for the observation that, with chronic administration of ketamine, higher doses may be required to obtain the therapeutic effect.

Little is known about whether tolerance can develop with ketamine or esketamine when it comes to their antidepressant effects. Unfortunately, none of the clinical studies to date have provided data to support or refute the possibility that repeated exposure to the same dose of ketamine produces tolerance, or sensitization, when it comes to antidepressant properties. This is important information to be had because tolerance could mean higher and higher doses would be needed to achieve antidepressant efficacy until it eventually becomes ineffective.

Effect of Repeated Ketamine Exposure on the Human Brain

To date, there is a limited amount of reliable information on how repeated use of ketamine can influence the function of the human brain. The few available studies indicate that frequent use of ketamine causes persistent impairments on memory.[12]

Clinical trials with repeated ketamine use have generally not yet employed brain imaging methods that can give us clues about how brain function may be affected after repeated use. Some such studies exist, though. One of these studies, performed in 2005, found changes in dopamine function in the brains of individuals who recreationally and regularly used ketamine. A major strength of the study was that the scanned subjects were not polydrug users, and thus the observed effects were likely associated only with repeated ketamine use. The researchers focused on dopamine function in the *prefrontal cortex*, a brain region responsible for high-order brain functions such as attention, reasoning, and decision-making, as well as emotional regulation. Dopamine function in these repeated ketamine users was found to be compromised in a manner that suggested it had become hypoactive.[13] While not conclusive, these findings do raise some concern because reduced activity of dopamine in the prefrontal cortex is associated with cognitive decline, such as impaired attention and decision-making capacity.

Ketamine and Suicide

Ketamine is currently in several clinical trials to determine its impact on suicidality. Given that untreated depression is strongly associated with suicide, ketamine can potentially have a lifesaving effect on individuals at imminent risk of suicide. Unfortunately, results of earlier trials of ketamine for suicide prevention were unconvincing at best because of low patient numbers and lack of placebo control. The following is a summary of one such trial, which was considered to be a "positive" trial: "Twelve subjects with treatment-resistant unipolar or bipolar major depression and suicidal ideation were given repeated (up to 6) thrice-weekly acute-phase intravenous infusions of ketamine. Five subjects who remitted during the acute-phase experienced further improvement during continuation-phase treatment. Four lost remission status during the post-continuation phase, but all were still classified as positive treatment responders. One subject developed behavioral outbursts and suicide threats during follow-up while hospitalized, and one subject died by suicide several weeks after the end of follow-up."[14]

In another study, often cited as evidence for the positive impact of ketamine on preventing suicide, the investigators gave ketamine to twenty-four individuals. Suicidal ideation was measured by how individuals answer a psychological questionnaire called the Beck Scale for Suicidal Ideation (BSI). This is a standard and reliable approach, based on data and ideas put forth in a landmark paper by Aaron Beck, Maria Kovacs, and Arlene Weisseman.[15] Using the BSI, it was found that ketamine after twenty-four hours had no positive effect. After forty-eight hours, the researchers reported a positive, but weak, effect. Moreover, all patients, including those that showed a positive response, had worsened by seven days after treatment.

Multiple placebo-controlled trials with esktamine are being completed as this book is being written, and results of those studies will be critical in shaping our future use of ketemine. So far, however, reports of increased rates of suicides days or weeks after the last dose of ketamine, which have been dismissed as not caused by ketamine, are disconcerting: What if relapse from ketamine or esketamine treatment leads to more intense symptoms and sustained or emerging suicidal thoughts for days and weeks?

The potential side effects may be more worrisome with esketamine versus racemic ketamine. Johnson & Johnson indicates in its published work that it chose to use multiple esketamine doses because there was a high degree of relapse with fewer treatments, necessitating twice or thrice weekly treatment with the drug.

There is a neuroplasticity phenomenon discovered by addiction researchers called *incubation*.[16] This refers to the observation that some of the adverse effects of the drug, including intense craving in addicts, become more intense days and weeks after the last exposure to the drug.[17] It is noteworthy that some cellular mechanisms that are attributed to Ketamine's antidepressant effects, such as activation of BDNF, are also seen during incubation from drugs of abuse.[18] Is there an incubation phenomenon associated with ketamine? If yes, are there detrimental effects of that incubation? Will relapses occur faster, requiring higher and more frequent doses of ketamine to treat symptoms? How high can we push the dose and the frequency of its administration before causing profound and irreversible neurotoxicity?

Adding to the concern is the problem of for-profit clinics "specializing" in off-label treatment use of ketamine, which have become more and more prevalent. These clinics use anecdotal testimonies from individual patients for marketing purposes but provide little if any data to the public, let alone in peer-reviewed journals, about the long-term impact on the individuals they have treated. It is not even clear that they collect the data related to suicide ideation or attempted suicides days or weeks after treatment—and even if they did, if they are obligated to report it.

7

WHERE DO WE GO FROM HERE?

Clinical Status of Ketamine

About fifteen years ago, Dutch medical historians Snelders, Kaplan, and Pieters coined the term *Seige cycle* to describe the dynamic phases of the career of psychiatric drugs. The term was named after Max Seige, a German psychiatrist who was the first to propose the concept that psychotropic drugs have a cyclical livelihood. The three phases of the Seige cycle are "initial enthusiasm and therapeutic optimism; subsequent negative appraisal; and finally, limited use."[1]

Ketamine is on track to follow this cycle (figure 9): currently, it is in its initial stage of generating remarkable enthusiasm as a novel antidepressant that can provide immediate relief to severely depressed patients and potentially work to prevent suicide. But approval of ketamine as an antidepressant has raised a number of concerns and

Stage 1 – The Hype Stage—The media, patients, and many physicians are enthusiastic about ketamine and optimistic that it will revolutionize treatment of depression.

Stage 2 – Negative Appraisal—Thrice weekly indefinite exposure to esketamine has unknown consequences. As ketamine and esketamine are used more frequently at the thrice weekly recommended doses for extensive period of time, there will be emergence of genitourinary and other serious side effects as well as potential drug withdrawal symptoms leading to abuse.

Stage 3 – Limited Use—With appreciation that the dangerous side effects are due to repeated use, intermittent use of ketamine would continue to be useful as an antidepressant when other treatments have failed.

Figure 9 Predicted stages of the career of ketamine as an antidepressant.

warnings from physicians and patient advocates because its path to approval for use in depression was unusually rapid. More importantly, there is virtually no long-term safety data about repeated use of ketamine or esketamine. The fact that now we are recommending that patients with treatment-resistant depression take these drugs twice or thrice weekly indefinitely causes concern given that we have little data about the impact of frequent, prolonged ketamine use on patients' health. Some studies suggest that there are several unpleasant and potentially fatal urogenital and hepatic consequences of chronic ketamine use. Based on the reported side effects of repeated illicit use of

There is virtually no long-term safety data about repeated use of ketamine or esketamine.

ketamine, potential for development of tolerance or abuse, and general lack of safety data on its long-term use, negative appraisal of ketamine may begin to emerge, reducing its use and popularity.

All drugs have side effects. Thus, while there is a keen sense that the renal and other potentially dangerous side effects of long-term use of ketamine or esketamine will be prohibitive to its use as a common antidepressant, limited use may remain beneficial and safe. Ketamine therefore is likely to end the Seige cycle as a useful drug for short-term use in some patients who have not responded to other modes of treatment.

Theory versus Data: Challenges of Studying Ketamine in the Laboratory

Regardless of the future clinical status of ketamine, the fact that a single dose can treat symptoms of depression within hours of being administered has turned antidepressant-focused laboratory research upside down.

Before this discovery, it was an accepted assumption that antidepressants take several weeks to work. Accordingly, the focus of laboratory-based research, mostly performed in rats and mice, was on studying how several weeks of exposure to an antidepressant can change the brain.

After the discovery of the antidepressant effects of ketamine, a large number of laboratory-based studies attempted to understand the mechanism of action of a single dose of ketamine on the same depression models that had been used to study the older antidepressant drugs. As described in chapter 6, these studies primarily focused on the theory that ketamine produces its antidepressant effects by blocking NMDA receptors. Multiple high-profile papers in influential journals, including *Nature* and *Science*, provided elegant data on molecular and cellular details of how ketamine could be acting as an antidepressant in rats and mice through mechanisms that directly or indirectly involved the NMDA receptor.

But no matter how convincing and elegant the data in rats and mice may be, one cannot argue with clinical trials. As reviewed in chapter 6, all clinical trials so far with drugs other than ketamine that work on the NMDA receptor directly or on downstream effects predicted by animal studies have failed to produce similar antidepressant activity as ketamine in humans. These have included at least four drugs. Three older ones (memantine, rislenemdaz, and lanicemine) and a new one (rapastinel) that directly or indirectly block the function of the NMDA receptor by different mechanisms have all failed in clinical trials. So have drugs that may mimic the downstream NMDA-receptor-blocking effects of ketamine. Does this suggest that we are going about studying the antidepressant effects of ketamine in the wrong way?

At least three approaches to studying ketamine in the laboratory have been problematic. The first is that we are relying on relatively arbitrary animal models to test the validity of our mechanisms. These animal models were designed from a primitive understanding of behavioral neuroscience in the 1950s. These models (discussed in chapter 6) typically involve exposing animals to chronic stress or to other manipulations, such as forcing them to swim, that presumably create a state of helplessness in the animal. These models, or *behavioral endpoints*, were successful in identifying drugs like tricyclic antidepressants and SSRIs, but they have since been unsuccessful for identifying novel antidepressants. Moreover, the whole point of studying ketamine is to find why it works differently than the old antidepressants,

By applying the old endpoints for studying antidepressants in the laboratory to ketamine, we limit our ability to understand its effects because we are showing a different mechanism to reach the same effect. But clinically, ketamine does not have the same effect as the older antidepressants. In particular, it works in patients that have *not* responded to the older drugs, thus making endpoint measures that worked with those drugs challenging to interpret.

The second problem of our approaches to studying ketamine in the laboratory has been difficulty studying its clinical time course of effect. Most of the proposed NMDA receptor–mediated mechanisms for its antidepressant effects involve so-called neuroplasticity, by which changes in protein levels, gene expression, and branching patterns of neurons become apparent about a day after exposure to ketamine and last indefinitely (at least in the brains of rodents). But the effects of ketamine, while apparent a few hours after exposure, last only a few days in humans. How then is a permanent or long-lasting effect in rodents relevant to short-lasting clinical effects of ketamine in humans? Few, if any, laboratory-based studies have identified mechanisms associated with ketamine that are consistent with its clinical time course of antidepressant effect.

Finally, laboratory studies often focus on molecular mechanisms that are broadly distributed and common to many brain systems. For example, nearly every brain region relies on glutamate receptor–mediated signaling as key hardware for synaptic circuitry. Even if researchers focus on a specific brain region, seldom is control data presented to show that the effect does (or does not) generalize to other brain regions. Human imaging studies have revealed that in patients with depression, ketamine produces a complex pattern of effect that is not global and is restricted to specific brain networks of individuals with depressive disorders.[2] Moreover, the effect of ketamine is highly dynamic and involves changes to *functional connectivity*, which refers to how interaction between brain regions dynamically changes to produce various brain states.[3] To move the field forward, brain-region-specific and state-dependent effects should be studied in animal models in the context of clinically relevant symptoms of depression.

Moving forward, it should be appreciated that ketamine's effects in the clinical setting may be difficult to model effectively. With traditional antidepressants, about 70 percent of patients respond, and these drugs are effective in "traditional" animal models of depressive behavior. Ketamine, by contrast, has been studied mostly in individuals unresponsive to traditional drugs, suggesting the pathophysiology of the symptoms may be quite distinct, both in degree and in kind, in individuals who respond to traditional antidepressants versus ketamine. More importantly, even in patients with treatment-resistant depression that have participated in recent clinical trials of ketamine, rates of positive response to ketamine lie between 10 and 50 percent, depending on the study in question. Even as we better understand ketamine's mechanism of action using rodent models, we must keep in mind that many factors determine its rapid but short-acting effectiveness in treating depression. Thus, any laboratory-defined mechanism of ketamine that is observed consistently in all animals may not be relevant to its antidepressant effects.

What Is Next? The Future of Fast-Acting Antidepressants

The genie is out of the bottle. The awareness that symptoms of depression can be alleviated quickly is making us rethink animal models and other approaches to design better antidepressant medications. Hopes for the design of newer and better antidepressants notwithstanding, ketamine may be the tip of the iceberg in our approach to use old drugs to rapidly treat symptoms of depression.

Recent studies using other old psychoactive drugs such as ecstasy and psychedelics like LSD and psilocybin (the active ingredient of magic mushrooms) are indicating that, similar to ketamine, a single dose of these drugs may help alleviate symptoms of depression and do so for much longer than the usual two to five days of relief produced by ketamine.

One of the first clinical studies related to this approach involved using psilocybin to assist with psychotherapy in treatment-resistant patients.[4] These were severely to moderately depressed patients who had been previously unresponsive to at least two other treatment methods, and had suffered from depression for an average of eighteen years. The study combined brain imaging and up to six months of follow-up. All patients showed improvement in their symptoms. This is much better than ketamine, which generally works on a subgroup of patients. The time course of effect also was quite different from ketamine. Improvement was apparent one week after treatment, with maximal effects seen at five weeks. More impressively, positive results remained evident at three and six months after the single treatment. The brain imaging studies showed lasting changes in the collaborative activity of some of the brain networks that are associated with mood and anxiety.[5]

This first study was relatively small, with only about twenty patients, and did not include a control group or placebo groups. But the results were impressive enough, especially since no adverse effects were reported by any of the patients, to warrant further research with psilocybin.

Several other studies followed up on the topic. A recent study providing a meta-analysis of published clinical trials of psilocybin in depressed patients provides a positive outlook: "Across four studies (one uncontrolled; three randomized, placebo-controlled; N = 117), within-group pre-post and pre-follow-up effects on anxiety and depression were large and statistically significant."[6]

These studies are obviously limited because they include small numbers of patients. In addition, in studies using profoundly psychoactive drugs such as psilocybin, it is difficult to have a proper placebo-controlled group. The same limitation, of course, applies to ketamine.

Despite these limitations, the impressively consistent and long-lasting therapeutic effects of this treatment combined with a general lack of side effects have led to the FDA and the European Medicines Agency (EMA; the regulatory agency responsible for safety regulation of the food and drug products in Europe) to approve a multicenter, multi-country trial of psilocybin. This study will be supported by the UK-based pharmaceutical company COMPASS Pathways. Another company, US-based Usona, is also gearing up to develop psilocybin for treatment of depression and other psychiatric illnesses.

The hope is that if the results of the current, more expansive clinical trials are positive, the FDA and EMA will approve psilocybin as a medicine for the benefits of patients with treatment-resistant depression. This will be a significant advance. Unlike ketamine, which was already approved for clinical use as an anesthetic before its antidepressant effects were discovered, psilocybin has been assigned a Schedule 1 status by the United States Drug Enforcement Administration (DEA). This classification is assigned to drugs with no currently accepted medical use and a high potential for abuse, making approval of the clinical use of psilocybin an uphill battle.

Conclusion

Even if emerging side effects dampen the current push to make ketamine available to patients, there remains excitement about this molecule as a scientific tool for understanding depression and rapidly relieving its symptoms.

Depression is a major cause of disability worldwide. According to the US Centers for Disease Control and Prevention, about one in ten adults suffer from mood disorders, including depression. If left untreated, depression can profoundly affect day-to-day functioning and quality of life. Depression is also deadly. It increases rates of diabetes and heart disease and is associated with significantly increased rates of suicide. Because ketamine works differently than traditional antidepressants, both by working quickly and by acting on potentially different brain mechanisms, it is fundamentally changing how clinicians think about treating depression and how laboratories study depression. This trend is likely to continue with the resurgence of other old psychoactive drugs, especially psilocybin, that, similar to ketamine, work to treat symptoms of treatment-resistant depression after a single dose.

Ketamine may be an old drug, and the enthusiastic acclaim for it as an antidepressant may be hyped, but it is forcing us to think outside the box about the biology of depression. This is cause for optimism because as in other maladies, such as cancer or HIV/AIDS, effective treatments—and ultimately, a cure—can only come from understanding the biology of the illness.

Ketamine may be an old drug, and the enthusiastic acclaim for it as an antidepressant may be hyped, but it is forcing us to think outside the box about the biology of depression.

ACKNOWLEDGMENTS

The bulk of this book is based on the knowledge that I have acquired over three decades of doing laboratory research with psychoactive drugs, including ketamine. I owe much of this knowledge to my mentors and teachers, who trained me as a chemist and a neuroscientist, and to my trainees and colleagues, who devoted their careers to studying the biology of brain illnesses. Among my colleagues, I am especially indebted to John Krystal, who first interested me in working with ketamine in the early 1990s when we were both assistant professors in the Department of Psychiatry at Yale.

Much of the content and organization of this book was developed through conversations with my family: Charles, Mazdak, and Anahita Bradberry. They are scientists and artists who constructively evaluated my ideas and helped me edit the text and the artwork in the book.

Finally, I must acknowledge the MIT Press team. They were delightful to work with and made all stages of this writing adventure much easier than I had anticipated.

GLOSSARY

Acetylcholine
A neurotransmitter molecule used by neurons in the central nervous system, as well as by neurons that activate muscles at the neuromuscular junction.

Affinity for a brain receptor
A measure reflecting the strength of interaction between a molecule and a receptor, reflecting the degree of binding that occurs at a given concentration.

Agonist
A molecule that when bound to a receptor, activates that receptor to produce a biological effect.

AMPA
Abbreviation for the chemical α-amino-3-hydroxy-5-methyl-4-isoxazolepropionic acid and the name of a subtype of glutamate receptor.

Analgesia
Drug-induced reduction in pain from a given stimulus.

Antagonist
A molecule that, when bound to a receptor, prevents the binding of an agonist that would normally produce a biological effect.

BDNF
Brain-derived neurotrophic factor.

CDC
Centers for Disease Control and Prevention.

Chirality
The structural nature of a molecule, enabling it to exist in two possible mirror images.

Dirty drug
A drug that acts on multiple proteins and has multiple mechanisms of action.

Dopamine
A neurotransmitter in the central nervous system, the loss of which results in Parkinson's disease, and which is broadly implicated in attention, memory, and drug reward.

ECT
Electroconvulsive therapy.

FDA
Food and Drug Administration.

Isomer
A subtype of molecule from a group that is defined by the same chemical formula. This can mean that it has a different branching structure, or it could be a chiral isomer in which it is the mirror image of the same molecule.

MDD
Major depressive disorder.

Meta-analysis
A type of statistical analysis in which data from multiple different studies are combined in order to achieve greater statistical power in determining an effect.

Neuron
The building block cells in the brain that are able to communicate with others, often at a distance by virtue of the electrical properties of its cell membrane.

Neuronal network
A group of neurons that act together to achieve a defined function. This often can occur across multiple parts of the brain acting in concert.

Neuropharmacology
The study of drugs that interact with the nervous system.

Neuropsychopharmacology
The study of drugs that interact with the nervous system and produce changes in behavior or mood or that alleviate a central nervous system–based disease state.

Neurotoxicity
An action or attribute that injures nervous system components.

Neurotransmission
The action in which one neuron communicates with another by releasing a neurotransmitter that binds to a receptor on that neuron to produce a change in its activity.

NMDA
N-methyl-D-aspartate.

Off-label
Medical use of an FDA-approved drug for a use that is not specifically approved by the FDA.

Organic chemistry
The branch of chemistry that studies carbon-containing compounds.

PCP
Hallucinogen drug phencyclidine, also known as angel dust.

Polymorphism
Variability in a gene that can sometimes produce differences in its function.

Receptor affinity
A measure of how strongly a receptor interacts with a given molecule. It indicates the fraction of receptors occupied as the concentration of that molecule increases.

Synapse
A point of contact between two brain cells.

Therapeutic index
A measure of drug safety. It is the ratio between the dose of a drug that causes harm and that which is therapeutic.

TRD
Treatment-resistant depression.

Tricyclics
A class of antidepressant drugs.

NOTES

Chapter 1

1. C. L. Stevens, "Aminiethones et leurs procedes de preparation," Belgium patent (1963).
2. V. H. Maddox, E. F. Godefroi, and R. F. Parcell, "The Synthesis of Phencyclidine and Other 1-Arylcyclohexylamines," *Journal of Medicinal Chemistry* 8 (1965): 230–235, https://doi.org/10.1021/jm00326a019.
3. G. R. Price, "New Drugs to Tune Up," *Popular Science* 173 (November 1958): 142–152, 250.
4. Maddox, Godefroi, and Parcell, "Synthesis of Phencyclidine."
5. E. F. Domino, "History and Pharmacology of PCP and PCP-Related Analogs," *Journal of Psychedelic Drugs* 12 (1980): 223–227, https://doi.org/10.1080/02791072.1980.10471430.
6. N. B. S. Denomme, "The Domino Effect: Ed Domino's Early Studies of Psychoactive Drugs," *Journal of Psychoactive Drugs* 50 (2018): 298–305, https://doi.org/10.1080/02791072.2018.1506599.
7. Denomme, "Domino Effect."
8. E. D. Luby, B. D. Cohen, G. Rosenbaum, J. S. Gottlieb, and R. Kelley, "Study of a New Schizophrenomimetic Drug: Sernyl," *AMA Archives of Neurology & Psychiatry* 81 (1959): 363–369, https://doi.org/10.1001/archneurpsyc.1959.02340150095011.
9. B. Moghaddam and J. H. Krystal, "Capturing the Angel in 'Angel Dust': Twenty Years of Translational Neuroscience Studies of NMDA Receptor Antagonists in Animals and Humans," *Schizophrenia Bulletin* 38 (2012): 942–949, https://doi.org/10.1093/schbul/sbs075.
10. Domino, "History and Pharmacology of PCP."
11. E. F. Domino, P. Chodoff, and G. Corssen, "Pharmacologic Effects of Ci-581, a New Dissociative Anesthetic, in Man," *Clinical Pharmacology & Therapeutics* 6 (1965): 279–291, https://doi.org/10.1002/cpt196563279.

Chapter 2

1. S. J. Mercer, "'The Drug of War'—A Historical Review of the Use of Ketamine in Military Conflicts," *Journal of the Royal Naval Medical Service* 95 (2009): 145–150.

2. J. Persson, "Ketamine in Pain Management," *CNS Neuroscience & Therapeutics* 19 (2013): 396–402, https://doi.org/10.1111/cns.12111.

3. G. Lenz and R. Stehle, "Anesthesia under Field Conditions: A Review of 945 Cases," *Acta Anaesthesiologica Scandinavica* 28 (1984): 351–356, https://doi.org/10.1111/j.1399-6576.1984.tb02075.x; S. J. Mercer, "'The Drug of War'—A Historical Review of the Use of Ketamine in Military Conflicts," *Journal of the Royal Naval Medical Service* 95 (2009): 145–150; R. Moy and C. Wright, "Ketamine for Military Prehospital Analgesia and Sedation in Combat Casualties," *Journal of the Royal Army Medical Corps* 164 (2018): 436–437, https://doi.org/10.1136/jramc-2018-000910.

4. S. A. Bergman, "Ketamine: Review of Its Pharmacology and Its Use in Pediatric Anesthesia," *Anesthesia Progress* 46 (1999): 10–20.

5. A. J. Mellor, "Anaesthesia in Austere Environments," *Journal of the Royal Army Medical Corps* 151 (2005): 272–276, https://doi.org/10.1136/jramc-151-04-09.

6. K. Hunt, "Boys Rescued from Thai Cave Were Sedated with Ketamine," CNN Health, April 4, 2019, https://www.cnn.com/2019/04/04/health/thailand-boys-cave-ketamine-intl/index.html.

7. M. Wright, "Pharmacologic Effects of Ketamine and Its Use in Veterinary Medicine," *Journal of the American Veteran Medical Association* 180 (1982): 1462–1471.

8. Persson, "Ketamine in Pain Management."

9. E. Soto, D. R. Stewart, A. J. Mannes, S. L. Ruppert, K. Baker, D. Zlott, et al., "Oral Ketamine in the Palliative Care Setting: A Review of the Literature and Case Report of a Patient with Neurofibromatosis Type 1 and Glomus Tumor-Associated Complex Regional Pain Syndrome," *American Journal of Hospice & Palliative Care* 29 (2012): 308–317, https://doi.org/10.1177/1049909111416345.

10. K. L. Jansen and R. Darracot-Cankovic, "The Nonmedical Use of Ketamine, Part Two: A Review of Problem Use and Dependence," *Journal of Psychoactive Drugs* 33 (2001): 151–158, https://doi.org/10.1080/02791072.2001.10400480; S. E. Lankenau and M. C. Clatts, "Drug Injection Practices among High-Risk Youths: The First Shot of Ketamine," *Journal of Urban Health* 81 (2004): 232–248, https://doi.org/10.1093/jurban/jth110; D. C. Ompad, S. Galea, C. M. Fuller, D. Phelan, and D. Vlahov, "Club Drug Use Among Minority Substance Users in New York City," *Journal of Psychoactive Drugs* 36 (2004): 397–399, https://doi.org/10.1080/02791072.2004.10400039.

11. C. M. Chang, T. L. Wu, T. T. Ting, C. Y. Chen, L. W. Su, and W. J. Chen, "Mis-anaesthetized Society: Expectancies and Recreational Use of Ketamine

in Taiwan," *BMC Public Health* 19 (2019): 1307, https://doi.org/10.1186/s12889-019-7616-1; W. C. Cheng and K. L. Dao, "Prevalence of Drugs of Abuse Found in Testing of Illicit Drug Seizures and Urinalysis of Selected Population in Hong Kong," *Forensic Science International* 299 (2019): 6–16, https://doi.org/10.1016/j.forsciint.2019.03.022.

12. C. E. Stewart, "Ketamine as a Street Drug," *Emergency Medical Service* 3034 (2001): 34; W. C. Cheng and K. L. Dao, "The Occurrence of Alcohol/Drugs by Toxicological Examination of Selected Drivers in Hong Kong," *Forensic Science International* 275 (2017): 242–253, https://doi.org/10.1016/j.forsciint.2017.03.022.

13. S. S. Yang, M. Y. Jang, K. H. Lee, W. T. Hsu, Y. C. Chen, W. S. Chen, et al., "Sexual and Bladder Dysfunction in Male Ketamine Abusers: A Large-Scale Questionnaire Study," *PLoS One* 13 (2018): e0207927, https://doi.org/10.1371/journal.pone.0207927; C. C. Li, S. T. Wu, T. L. Cha, G. H Sun, D. S. Yu, and E. Meng, "A Survey for Ketamine Abuse and Its Relation to the Lower Urinary Tract Symptoms in Taiwan," *Scientific Reports* 9 (2019): 7240, https://doi.org/10.1038/s41598-019-43746-x.

14. R. R. Sircar, H. Samaan, R. Nichtenhauser, L. D. Snell, K. M. Johnson, J. Rivier, et al., "Modulation of Brain NMDA Receptors: Common Mechanism of Sigma/PCP Receptors and Their Exogenous and Endogenous Ligands," *NIDA Research Monograph* 75 (1986): 157–160.

15. E. D. Luby, B. D. Cohen, G. Rosenbaum, J. S. Gottlieb, and R. Kelley, "Study of a New Schizophrenomimetic Drug; Sernyl," *AMA Archives of Neurology and Psychiatry* 81 (1959): 363–369, https://doi.org/10.1001/archneurpsyc.1959.02340150095011.

16. B. Moghaddam, "Recent Basic Findings in Support of Excitatory Amino Acid Hypotheses of Schizophrenia," *Progress in Neuropsychopharmacology and Biological Psychiatry* 18 (1994): 859–870, https://doi.org/10.1016/0278-5846(94)90102-3; B. Moghaddam and B. W. Adams, "Reversal of Phencyclidine Effects by a Group II Metabotropic Glutamate Receptor Agonist in Rats," *Science* 281 (1998): 1349–1352, https://doi.org/10.1126/science.281.5381.1349; J. T. Coyle, "The Glutamatergic Dysfunction Hypothesis for Schizophrenia," *Harvard Review of Psychiatry* 3 (1996): 241–253, https://doi.org/10.3109/10673229609017192; J. T. Coyle, "The Nagging Question of the Function of N-acetylaspartylglutamate," *Neurobiology of Disease* 4 (1997): 231–238, https://doi.org/10.1006/nbdi.1997.0153; D. C. Javitt and S. R. Zukin, "Recent Advances in the Phencyclidine Model of Schizophrenia," *American Journal of Psychiatry* 148 (1991): 1301–1308, https://doi.org/10.1176/ajp.148.10.1301; E. Leiderman, I. Zylberman, S. R. Zukin, T. B. Cooper, and D. C. Javitt,

"Preliminary Investigation of High-Dose Oral Glycine on Serum Levels and Negative Symptoms in Schizophrenia: An Open-Label Trial," *Biological Psychiatry* 39 (1996): 213–215, https://doi.org/10.1016/0006-3223(95)00585-4.
17. J. H. Krystal, L. P. Karper, J. P. Seibyl, G. K. Freeman, R. Delaney, J. D. Bremner, et al., "MDSubanesthetic Effects of the Noncompetitive NMDA Antagonist, Ketamine, in Humans: Psychotomimetic, Perceptual, Cognitive, and Neuroendocrine Responses," *Archives of General Psychiatry* 51 (1994): 199–214, https://doi.org/10.1001/archpsyc.1994.03950030035004.
18. B. Moghaddam, B. Adams, A. Verma, and D. Daly, "Activation of Glutamatergic Neurotransmission by Ketamine: A Novel Step in the Pathway from NMDA Receptor Blockade to Dopaminergic and Cognitive Disruptions Associated with the Prefrontal Cortex," *Journal of Neuroscience* 17 (1997): 2921–2927.
19. R. M. Berman, A. Cappiello, A. Anand, D. A. Oren, G. R. Heninger, D. S. Charney, and J. H. Krystal, "Antidepressant Effects of Ketamine in Depressed Patients," *Biological Psychiatry* 47 (2000): 351–354, https://doi.org/10.1016/s0006-3223(99)00230-9.

Chapter 3

1. E. R. Kandel and S. Mack, *Principles of Neural Science* (New York: McGraw Hill, 2014).
2. Z. L. Kruk and C. J. Pycock, *Neurotransmitters and Drugs* (London: Chapman & Hill, 1991).
3. K. Hashimoto, "Rapid-Acting Antidepressant Ketamine, Its Metabolites and Other Candidates: A Historical Overview and Future Perspective," *Psychiatry and Clinical Neurosciences* 73 (2019): 613–627, https://doi.org/10.1111/pcn.12902.
4. D. Lodge, N. A. Anis, and N. R. Burton, "Effects of Optical Isomers of Ketamine on Excitation of Cat and Rat Spinal Neurones by Amino Acids and Acetylcholine," *Neuroscience Letters* 29 (1982): 281–286, https://doi.org/10.1016/0304-3940(82)90330-5; B. L. Roth, S. Gibbons, W. Arunotayanun, X. P. Huang, V. Setola, R. Treble, and L. Iversen, "The Ketamine Analogue Methoxetamine and 3- and 4-Methoxy Analogues of Phencyclidine Are High Affinity and Selective Ligands for the Glutamate NMDA Receptor," *PLoS One* 8 (2013): e59334, https://doi.org/10.1371/journal.pone.0059334.
5. S. Nakanishi, "Molecular Diversity of Glutamate Receptors and Implications for Brain Function," *Science* 258 (1992): 597–603, https://doi.org/10.1126/science.1329206.
6. Roth et al., "Ketamine Analogue Methoxetamine."

7. B. Moghaddam, B. Adams, A. Verma, and D. Daly, "Activation of Glutamatergic Neurotransmission by Ketamine: A Novel Step in the Pathway from NMDA Receptor Blockade to Dopaminergic and Cognitive Disruptions Associated with the Prefrontal Cortex," *Journal of Neuroscience* 17 (1997): 2921–2927; M. E. Jackson, H. Homayoun, and B. Moghaddam, "NMDA Receptor Hypofunction Produces Concomitant Firing Rate Potentiation and Burst Activity Reduction in the Prefrontal Cortex," *Proceedings of the National Academy of Sciences of the United States of America* 101 (2004): 8467–8472, https://doi.org/10.1073/pnas.0308455101; H. Homayoun and B. Moghaddam, "NMDA Receptor Hypofunction Produces Opposite Effects on Prefrontal Cortex Interneurons and Pyramidal Neurons," *Journal of Neuroscience* 27 (2007): 11496–11500, https://doi.org/10.1523/jneurosci.2213-07.2007.

8. A. Nikiforuk, T. Kos, M. Holuj, A. Potasiewicz, and P. Popik, "Positive Allosteric Modulators of Alpha 7 Nicotinic Acetylcholine Receptors Reverse Ketamine-Induced Schizophrenia-like Deficits in Rats," *Neuropharmacology* 101 (2016): 389–400, https://doi.org/10.1016/j.neuropharm.2015.07.034.

9. S. Kapur and P. Seeman, "NMDA Receptor Antagonists Ketamine and PCP Have Direct Effects on the Dopamine D(2) and Serotonin 5-HT(2) Receptors-Implications for Models of Schizophrenia," *Molecular Psychiatry* 7 (2002): 837–844, https://doi.org/10.1038/sj.mp.4001093; Roth et al., "Ketamine Analogue Methoxetamine."

10. K. Hirota, H. Okawa, B. L. Appadu, D. K. Grandy, L. A. Devi, and D. G. Lambert, "Stereoselective Interaction of Ketamine with Recombinant Mu, Kappa, and Delta Opioid Receptors Expressed in Chinese Hamster Ovary Cells," *Anesthesiology* 90 (1999): 174–182, https://doi.org/10.1097/00000542-199901000-00023; Roth et al., "Ketamine Analogue Methoxetamine."

11. N. R. Williams, B. D. Heifets, B. S. Bentzley, C. Blasey, K. D. Sudheimer, J. Hawkins, et al., "Attenuation of Antidepressant and Antisuicidal Effects of Ketamine by Opioid Receptor Antagonism," *Molecular Psychiatry* 24 (2019): 1779–1786, https://doi.org/10.1038/s41380-019-0503-4.

12. M. F. Ho, C. Correia, J. N. Ingle, R. Kaddurah-Daouk, L. Wang, S. H. Kaufmann, and R. M. Weinshilboum, "Ketamine and Ketamine Metabolites as Novel Estrogen Receptor Ligands: Induction of Cytochrome P450 and AMPA Glutamate Receptor Gene Expression," *Biochemical Pharmacology* 152 (2018): 279–292, https://doi.org/10.1016/j.bcp.2018.03.032.

13. M. Nishimura and K. Sato, "Ketamine Stereoselectively Inhibits Rat Dopamine Transporter," *Neuroscience Letters* 274 (1999): 131–134, https://doi.org/10.1016/s0304-3940(99)00688-6; Roth et al., "Ketamine Analogue Methoxetamine."

14. G. F. Gutierrez Aguilar, I. Alquisiras-Burgos, M. Espinoza-Rojo, and P. Aguilera, "Glial Excitatory Amino Acid Transporters and Glucose Incorporation," *Advances in Neurobiology* 16 (2017): 269–282, https://doi.org/10.1007/978-3-319-55769-4_13.

15. Y. Wang, L. Xie, C. Gao, L. Zhai, N. Zhang, and L. Guo, "Astrocytes Activation Contributes to the Antidepressant-like Effect of Ketamine but Not Acopolamine," *Pharmacology Biochemistry and Behavior* 170 (2018): 1–8, https://doi.org/10.1016/j.pbb.2018.05.001; Y. Hayashi, K. Kawaji, L. Sun, X. Zhang, K. Koyano, T. Yokoyama, et al., "H.Microglial Ca(2+)-Activated K(+) Channels Are Possible Molecular Targets for the Analgesic Effects of S-Ketamine on Neuropathic Pain," *Journal of Neuroscience* 31 (2011): 17370–17382, https://doi.org/10.1523/jneurosci.4152-11.2011.

16. P. Zanos, R. Moaddel, P. J. Morris, L. M. Riggs, J. N. Highland, P. Georgiou, et al., "Ketamine and Ketamine Metabolite Pharmacology: Insights into Therapeutic Mechanisms," *Pharmacological Reviews* 70 (2018): 621–660, https://doi.org/10.1124/pr.117.015198.

17. G. L. Collingridge, Y. Lee, Z. A. Bortolotto, H. Kang, and D. Lodge, "Antidepressant Actions of Ketamine Versus Hydroxynorketamine," *Biological Psychiatry* 81 (2017): e65–e67, https://doi.org/10.1016/j.biopsych.2016.06.029; P. Zanos, R. Moaddel, P. J. Morris, P. Georgiou, J. Fischell, G. Elmer, et al., "NMDAR Inhibition-Independent Antidepressant Actions of Ketamine Metabolites," *Nature* 533 (2016): 481–486, https://doi.org/10.1038/nature17998.

18. Y. Li, K. A. Jackson, B. Slon, J. R. Hardy, M. Franco, L. William, et al., "CYP2B6*6 Allele and Age Substantially Reduce Steady-State Ketamine Clearance in Chronic Pain Patients: Impact on Adverse Effects," *British Journal of Clinical Pharmacology* 80 (2015): 276–284, https://doi.org/10.1111/bcp.12614.

19. X. Pan, X. Zeng, J. Hong, C. Yuan, L. Cui, J. Ma, et al., "Effects of Ketamine on Metabolomics of Serum and Urine in Cynomolgus Macaques (Macaca fascicularis)," *Journal of the American Association for Laboratory Animal Science* 55 (2016): 558–564.

20. B. E. Hetzler, and B. S. Wautlet, "Ketamine-Induced Locomotion in Rats in an Open-Field," *Pharmacology Biochemistry and Behavior* 22 (1985): 653–655, https://doi.org/10.1016/0091-3057(85)90291-6.

21. A. M. Young and J. H. Woods, "Maintenance of Behavior by Ketamine and Related Compounds in Rhesus Monkeys with Different Self-Administration Histories," *Journal of Pharmacology and Experimental Therapeutics* 218 (1981): 720–727.

22. J. H. Krystal, L. P. Karper, J. P. Seibyl, G. K. Freeman, R. Delaney, J. D. Bremner, et al., "Subanesthetic Effects of the Noncompetitive NMDA Antagonist, Ketamine, in Humans: Psychotomimetic, Perceptual, Cognitive, and Neuroendocrine Responses," *Archives of General Psychiatry* 51 (1994): 199–214, https://doi.org/10.1001/archpsyc.1994.03950030035004; B. Moghaddam and D. Javitt, "From Revolution to Evolution: The Glutamate Hypothesis of Schizophrenia and Its Implication for Treatment," *Neuropsychopharmacology* 37 (2012): 4–15, https://doi.org/10.1038/npp.2011.181.
23. A. Y. Onaolapo, O. J. Ayeni, M. O. Ogundeji, A. Ajao, O. Onaolapo, A. R. Owolabi, "Subchronic Ketamine Alters Behaviour, Metabolic Indices and Brain Morphology in Adolescent Rats: Involvement of Oxidative Stress, Glutamate Toxicity and Caspase-3-Mediated Apoptosis," *Journal of Chemical Neuroanatomy* 96 (2019): 22–33, https://doi.org/10.1016/j.jchemneu.2018.12.002.
24. K. A. Trujillo and C. Y. Heller, "Ketamine Sensitization: Influence of Dose, Environment, Social Isolation and Treatment Interval," *Behavioural Brain Research* 378 (2020): 112271, https://doi.org/10.1016/j.bbr.2019.112271.
25. S. A. Gerb, J. E. Cook, A. E. Gochenauer, C. S. Young, L. K. Fulton, A. W. Grady, and K. B. Freeman, "Ketamine Tolerance in Sprague-Dawley Rats after Chronic Administration of Ketamine, Morphine, or Cocaine," *Comparative Medicine* 69 (2019): 29–34, https://doi.org/10.30802/aalas-cm-18-000053.
26. J. H. Krystal, A. Bennett, D. Abi-Saab, A. Belger, L. P. Karper, D. C. D'Souza, et al., "Dissociation of Ketamine Effects on Rule Acquisition and Rule Implementation: Possible Relevance to NMDA Receptor Contributions to Executive Cognitive Functions," *Biological Psychiatry* 47 (2000), 137–143, https://doi.org/10.1016/s0006-3223(99)00097-9.
27. C. F. Lanning and M. H. Harmel, "Ketamine Anesthesia," *Annual Review of Medicine* 26 (1975): 137–141, https://doi.org/10.1146/annurev.me.26.020175.001033.
28. X. Ke, Y. Ding, K. Xu, H. He, D. Wang, X. Deng, *et al.*, "The Profile of Cognitive Impairments in Chronic Ketamine Users," *Psychiatry Research* 266 (2018): 124–131, https://doi.org/10.1016/j.psychres.2018.05.050; P. J. Uhlhaas, I. Millard, L. Muetzelfeldt, H. V. Curran, and C. J. Morgan, "Perceptual Organization in Ketamine Users: Preliminary Evidence of Deficits on Night of Drug Use but Not 3 Days Later," *Journal of Psychopharmacology* 21 (2007): 347–352, https://doi.org/10.1177/0269881107077739.
29. R. Edward Roberts, H. V. Curran, K. J. Friston, and C. J. Morgan, "Abnormalities in White Matter Microstructure Associated with Chronic Ketamine Use," *Neuropsychopharmacology* 39 (2014): 329–338, https://doi.org/10.1038/npp.2013.195.

Chapter 4

1. D. P. Cantwell et al., *Diagnostic and Statistical Manual of Mental Disorders*, 3rd ed. (Washington, DC: American Psychiatric Association, 1981).

2. R. Burton and A. Gowland, *The Anatomy of Melancholy* (London: Penguin, 2019).

3. Z. Wang, X. Ma, and C. Xiao, "Standardized Treatment Strategy for Depressive Disorder," *Advances in Experimental Medicine and Biology* 1180 (2019): 193–199, https://doi.org/10.1007/978-981-32-9271-0_10.

4. R. B. Haukaas, I. B. Gjerde, G. Varting, H. E. Hallan, and S. Solem, "A Randomized Controlled Trial Comparing the Attention Training Technique and Mindful Self-Compassion for Students with Symptoms of Depression and Anxiety," *Frontiers in Psychology* 9 (2018): 827, https://doi.org/10.3389/fpsyg.2018.00827.

5. R. W. Lam, D. D. Wan, N. L. Cohen, and S. H. Kennedy, "Combining Antidepressants for Treatment-Resistant Depression: A Review," *Journal of Clinical Psychiatry* 63 (2002): 685–693, https://doi.org/10.4088/jcp.v63n0805.

6. M. Nasser, A. Tibi, and E. Savage-Smith, "Ibn Sina's Canon of Medicine: 11th Century Rules for Assessing the Effects of drugs," *Journal of the Royal Society of Medicine* 102 (2009): 78–80.

7. V. Bégaudeau, *Laudanum* (Paris: Books on Demand, 2015).

8. W. K. Summers, E. Robins, and T. Reich, "The Natural History of Acute Organic Mental Syndrome after Bilateral Electroconvulsive Therapy," *Biological Psychiatry* 14 (1979): 905–912.

9. C. H. Kellner, *Handbook of ECT* (Washington, DC: American Psychiatric Press, 1997).

10. P. Sinha, R. V. Reddy, P. Srivastava, U. M. Mehta, and R. D. Bharath, "Network Neurobiology of Electroconvulsive Therapy in Patients with Depression," *Psychiatry Research: Neuroimaging* 287 (2019): 31–40, https://doi.org/10.1016/j.pscychresns.2019.03.008.

11. T. A. Ban, "Fifty Years Chlorpromazine: A Historical Perspective," *Neuropsychiatric Disease and Treatment* 3 (2007): 495–500.

12. F. M. Berger, "Meprobamate: Its Pharmacologic Properties and Clinical Uses," *International Record of Medicine and General Practice Clinics* 169 (1956): 184–196.

13. J. L. McCartney, "A Nearly Fatal Reaction to Deprol," *JAMA* 194 (1965): 569–570.

14. C. F. McCarthy and M. R. Sheridan, "Hepatic Necrosis Due to Marsilid," *Gut* 1 (1960): 169–170.

15. R. Kuhn, "The Treatment of Depressive States with G 22355 (Imipramine Hydrochloride)," *American Journal of Psychiatry* 115 (1958): 459–464, https://doi.org/10.1176/ajp.115.5.459; H. Azima and R. H. Vispo, "Imipramine: A Potent New Anti-depressant Compound," *American Journal of Psychiatry* 115 (1958): 245–246, https://doi.org/10.1176/ajp.115.3.245.
16. J. Angst and W. Theobald, *Tofranil (imipramine)* (Bern: Stampfli, 1970).
17. R. Tissot, "The Common Pathophysiology of Monaminergic Psychoses: A New Hypothesis," *Neuropsychobiology* 1 (1975): 243–260, https://doi.org/10.1159/000117498.
18. A. Carlsson, "A Paradigm Shift in Brain Research," *Science* 294 (2001): 1021–1024, https://doi.org/10.1126/science.1066969.
19. R. W. Fuller, K. W. Perry, and B. B. Molloy, "Effect of an Uptake Inhibitor on Serotonin Metabolism in Rat Brain: Studies with 3-(p-trifluoromethylphenoxy)-N-methyl-3-phenylpropylamine (Lilly 110140)," *Life Sciences* 15 (1974): 1161–1171, https://doi.org/10.1016/s0024-3205(74)80012-3.
20. E. Wurtzel, *Prozac Nation* (New York: Riverhead Books, 2014).
21. P. L. Delgado, D. S. Charney, L. H. Price, G. K. Aghajanian, H. Landis, and G. R. Heninger, "Serotonin Function and the Mechanism of Antidepressant Action: Reversal of Antidepressant-Induced Remission by Rapid Depletion of Plasma Tryptophan," *Archives of General Psychiatry* 47 (1990): 411–418, https://doi.org/10.1001/archpsyc.1990.01810170011002.
22. P. L. Delgado, L. H. Price, H. L. Miller, R. M. Salomon, G. K. Aghajanian, G. R. Heninger, and D. S. Charney, "Serotonin and the Neurobiology of Depression: Effects of Tryptophan Depletion in Drug-Free Depressed Patients," *Archives of General Psychiatry* 51 (1994): 865–874, https://doi.org/10.1001/archpsyc.1994.03950110025005.
23. R. M. Sapolsky, "McEwen-Induced Modulation of Endocrine History: A Partial Review," *Stress* 2 (1997): 1–12, https://doi.org/10.3109/10253899709014733.
24. B. S. McEwen, "Central Effects of Stress Hormones in Health and Disease: Understanding the Protective and Damaging Effects of Stress and Stress Mediators," *European Journal of Pharmacology* 583 (2008): 174–185, https://doi.org/10.1016/j.ejphar.2007.11.071.
25. M. A. Smith, S. Makino, R. Kvetnansky, and R. M. Post, "Effects of Stress on Neurotrophic Factor Expression in the Rat Brain," *Annals of the New York Academy of Sciences* 771 (1995): 234–239, https://doi.org/10.1111/j.1749-6632.1995.tb44684.x.
26. M. Nibuya, S. Morinobu, and R. S. Duman, "Regulation of BDNF and trkB mRNA in Rat Brain by Chronic Electroconvulsive Seizure and Antidepressant Drug Treatments," *Journal of Neurosciences* 15 (1995): 7539–7547.

27. R. S. Duman, "Neurobiology of Stress, Depression, and Rapid Acting Antidepressants: Remodeling Synaptic Connections," *Depression and Anxiety* 31 (2014): 291–296, https://doi.org/10.1002/da.22227.
28. P. V. Nunes, C. F. Nascimento, H. K. Kim, A. C. Andreazza, H. P. Brentani, C. K. Suemoto, et al., "Low Brain-Derived Neurotrophic Factor Levels in Post-Mortem Brains of Older Adults with Depression and Dementia in a Large Clinicopathological Sample," *Journal of Affective Disorders* 241 (2018): 176–181, https://doi.org/10.1016/j.jad.2018.08.025.
29. S. Cahalan, *Brain on Fire: My Month of Madness* (Eastbourne, UK: Gardners Books, 2012).
30. J. H. Krystal, L. P. Karper, J. P. Seibyl, G. K. Freeman, R. Delaney, J. D. Bremner, et al., "Subanesthetic Effects of the Noncompetitive NMDA Antagonist, Ketamine, in Humans: Psychotomimetic, Perceptual, Cognitive, and Neuroendocrine Responses," *Archives of General Psychiatry* 51 (1994): 199–214, https://doi.org/10.1001/archpsyc.1994.03950030035004.
31. C. A. Zarate Jr., J. B. Singh, P. J. Carlson, N. E. Brutsche, R. Ameli, D. A. Luckenbaugh, et al., "A Randomized Trial of an N-methyl-D-aspartate Antagonist in Treatment-Resistant Major Depression," *Archives of General Psychiatry* 63 (2006): 856–864, https://doi.org/10.1001/archpsyc.63.8.856.
32. C. Yang, J. Yang, A. Luo, and K. Hashimoto, "Molecular and Cellular Mechanisms Underlying the Antidepressant Effects of Ketamine Enantiomers and Its Metabolites," *Translational Psychiatry* 9 (2019): 280, https://doi.org/10.1038/s41398-019-0624-1.
33. F. X. Vollenweider, K. L. Leenders, I. Oye, D. Hell, and J. Angst, "Differential Psychopathology and Patterns of Cerebral Glucose Utilisation Produced by (*S*)- and (*R*)-Ketamine in Healthy Volunteers Using Positron Emission Tomography (PET)," *European Neuropsychopharmacology* 7 (1997): 25–38, https://doi.org/10.1016/s0924-977x(96)00042-9.

Chapter 5

1. N. Li, B. Lee, R. J. Liu, M. Banasr, J. M. Dwyer, M. Iwata, et al., "mTOR-dependent Synapse Formation Underlies the Rapid Antidepressant Effects of NMDA Antagonists," *Science* 329 (2010): 959–964, https://doi.org/10.1126/science.1190287.
2. B. Moghaddam, B. Adams, A. Verma, and D. Daly, "Activation of Glutamatergic Neurotransmission by Ketamine: A Novel Step in the Pathway from NMDA Receptor Blockade to Dopaminergic and Cognitive Disruptions Associated with the Prefrontal Cortex," *Journal of Neuroscience* 17 (1997): 2921–2927.

3. J. H. Krystal, C. G. Abdallah, G. Sanacora, D. S. Charney, and R. S. Duman, "Ketamine: A Paradigm Shift for Depression Research and Treatment," *Neuron* 101 (2019): 774–778, https://doi.org/10.1016/j.neuron.2019.02.005.
4. R. N. Moda-Sava, M. H. Murdock, P. K. Parekh1, R. N. Fetcho1, B. S. Huang, and T. N. Huynh, "Sustained Rescue of Prefrontal Circuit Dysfunction by Antidepressant-Induced Spine Formation," *Science* 364 (2019): https://science.sciencemag.org/content/364/6436/eaat8078.
5. B. Moghaddam, "Stress Preferentially Increases Extraneuronal Levels of Excitatory Amino Acids in the Prefrontal Cortex: Comparison to Hippocampus and Basal Ganglia," *Journal of Neurochemistry* 60 (1993): 1650–1657, https://doi.org/10.1111/j.1471-4159.1993.tb13387.x.
6. A. E. Autry, M. Adachi, E. Nosyreva, E. S. Na, M. F. Los, P. F. Cheng, et al., "NMDA Receptor Blockade at Rest Triggers Rapid Behavioural Antidepressant Responses," *Nature* 475 (2011): 91–95, https://doi.org/10.1038/nature10130.
7. P. Zanos, R. Moaddel, P. J. Morris, P. Georgiou, J. Fischell, G. I. Elmer, et al., "NMDAR Inhibition-Independent Antidepressant Actions of Ketamine Metabolites," *Nature* 533 (2016): 481–486, https://doi.org/10.1038/nature17998.
8. M. Li., M. Woelfer, L. Colic, A. Safron, C. Chang, H. J. Heinze, et al., "Default Mode Network Connectivity Change Corresponds to Ketamine's Delayed Glutamatergic Effects," *European Archives of Psychiatry and Clinical Neuroscience* (2018), https://doi.org/10.1007/s00406-018-0942-y.
9. R. P. Lawson, C. L. Nord, B. Seymour, D. L. Thomas, P. Dayan, S. Pilling, et al., "Disrupted Habenula Function in Major Depression," *Molecular Psychiatry* 22 (2017): 202–208, https://doi.org/10.1038/mp.2016.81.
10. Y. Yang, Y. Cui, K. Sang, Y. Dong, Z. Ni, S. Ma, et al., "Ketamine Blocks Bursting in the Lateral Habenula to Rapidly Relieve Depression," *Nature* 554 (2018): 317–322, https://doi.org/10.1038/nature25509.
11. T. Kishimoto, J. M. Chawla, K. Hagi, C. A. Zarate, J. M. Kane, M. Bauer, et al., "Single-Dose Infusion Ketamine and Non-ketamine N-methyl-d-aspartate Receptor Antagonists for Unipolar and Bipolar Depression: A Meta-analysis of Efficacy, Safety and Time Trajectories," *Psychological Medicine* 46 (2016): 1459–1472, https://doi.org/10.1017/s0033291716000064.
12. T. Kato and R. S. Duman, "Rapastinel, a Novel Glutamatergic Agent with Ketamine-like Antidepressant Actions: Convergent Mechanisms," *Pharmacology Biochemistry and Behavior* 188 (2020): 172827, https://doi.org/10.1016/j.pbb.2019.172827.
13. C. G. Abdallah, L. A. Averill, R. Gueorguieva, S. Goktas, P. Purohit, M. Ranganathan, et al., "Rapamycin, an Immunosuppressant and mTORC1 Inhibitor, Triples the Antidepressant Response Rate of Ketamine at 2 Weeks Following

Treatment: A Double-Blind, Placebo-Controlled, Cross-Over, Randomized Clinical Trial," bioRXiv, https://www.biorxiv.org/content/10.1101/500959v1.
14. B. Beilin, Y. Rusabrov, Y. Shapira, L. Roytblat, L. Greemberg, I. Z. Yardeni, et al., "Low-Dose Ketamine Affects Immune Responses in Humans during the Early Postoperative Period," *British Journal of Anaesthesia* 99 (2007): 522–527, https://doi.org/10.1093/bja/aem218.
15. M. H. Chen, C. T. Li, W. C. Lin, C. J. Hong, P. C. Tu, Y. M. Bai, et al., "Rapid Inflammation Modulation and Antidepressant Efficacy of a Low-Dose Ketamine Infusion in Treatment-Resistant Depression: A Randomized, Double-Blind Control Study," *Psychiatry Research* 269 (2018): 207–211, https://doi.org/10.1016/j.psychres.2018.08.078.
16. M. Clarke, S. Razmjou, N. Prowse, Z. Dwyer, D. Litteljohn, R. Pentz, et al., "Ketamine Modulates Hippocampal Neurogenesis and Pro-inflammatory Cytokines but Not Stressor Induced Neurochemical Changes," *Neuropharmacology* 112 (2017): 210–220, https://doi.org/10.1016/j.neuropharm.2016.04.021.
17. M. F. Ho, C. Correia, J. N. Ingle, R. Kaddurah-Daouk, L. Wang, S. H. Kaufmann, et al., "Ketamine and Ketamine Metabolites as Novel Estrogen Receptor Ligands: Induction of Cytochrome P450 and AMPA Glutamate Receptor Gene Expression," *Biochemical Pharmacology* 152 (2018): 279–292, https://doi.org/10.1016/j.bcp.2018.03.032.
18. N. R. Williams, B. D. Heifets, B. S. Bentzley, C. Blasey, K. D. Sudheimer, J. Hawkins, et al., "Attenuation of Antidepressant and Antisuicidal Effects of Ketamine by Opioid Receptor Antagonism," *Molecular Psychiatry* 24 (2019): 1779–1786, https://doi.org/10.1038/s41380-019-0503-4.
19. G. Kheirabadi, M. Vafaie, D. Kheirabadi, Z. Mirlouhi, and R. Hajiannasab, "Comparative Effect of Intravenous Ketamine and Electroconvulsive Therapy in Major Depression: A Randomized Controlled Trial," *Advanced Biomedical Research* 8 (2019): 25, https://doi.org/10.4103/abr.abr_166_18.

Chapter 6

1. E. H. Turner, "Esketamine for Treatment-Resistant Depression: Seven Concerns about Efficacy and FDA Approval," *Lancet Psychiatry* 6 (2019): 977–979, https://doi.org/10.1016/s2215-0366(19)30394-3.
2. R. M. Berman, A. Cappiello, A. Anand, D. A. Oren, G. R. Heninger, D. S. Charney, et al., "Antidepressant Effects of Ketamine in Depressed Patients," *Biological Psychiatry* 47 (2000): 351–354, https://doi.org/10.1016/s0006-3223(99)00230-9.
3. C. M. Canuso, J. B. Singh, M. Fedgchin, L. Alphs, R. Lane, P. Lim, et al., "Efficacy and Safety of Intranasal Esketamine for the Rapid Reduction of Symptoms

of Depression and Suicidality in Patients at Imminent Risk for Suicide: Results of a Double-Blind, Randomized, Placebo-Controlled Study," *American Journal of Psychiatry* 175 (2018): 620–630, https://doi.org/10.1176/appi.ajp.2018.17060720.

4. J. L. Phillips, S. Norris, J. Talbot, T. Hatchard, A. Ortiz, M. Birmingham, et al., "Single and Repeated Ketamine Infusions for Reduction of Suicidal Ideation in Treatment-Resistant Depression," *Neuropsychopharmacology* (2019), https://doi.org/10.1038/s41386-019-0570-x.

5. Y. Li, R. Shen, G. Wen, R. Ding, A. Du, J. Zhou, et al., "Effects of Ketamine on Levels of Inflammatory Cytokines IL-6, IL-1beta, and TNF-alpha in the Hippocampus of Mice Following Acute or Chronic Administration," *Frontiers in Pharmacology* 8 (2017): 139, https://doi.org/10.3389/fphar.2017.00139.

6. M. L. S. Bates and K. A. Trujillo, "Long-Lasting Effects of Repeated Ketamine Administration in Adult and Adolescent Rats," *Behavioural Brain Research* 369 (2019): 111928, https://doi.org/10.1016/j.bbr.2019.111928; L. Sun, Q. Li, Q. Li, Y. Zhang, D. Liu, H. Jiang, et al., "Chronic Ketamine Exposure Induces Permanent Impairment of Brain Functions in Adolescent Cynomolgus Monkeys," *Addiction Biology* 19 (2014): 185–194, https://doi.org/10.1111/adb.12004.

7. L. R. Nagy, R. E. Featherstone, C. G. Hahn, and S. J. Siegel, "Delayed Emergence of Behavioral and Electrophysiological Effects Following Juvenile Ketamine Exposure in Mice," *Translational Psychiatry* 5 (2015): e635, https://doi.org/10.1038/tp.2015.111.

8. K. L. Jansen and R. Darracot-Cankovic, "The Nonmedical Use of Ketamine, Part Two: A Review of Problem Use and Dependence," *Journal of Psychoactive Drugs* 33 (2001): 151–158, https://doi.org/10.1080/02791072.2001.10400480.

9. K. W. Chan, T. M. Lee, A. M. Siu, D. P. Wong, C. M. Kam, S. K. Tsang, et al., "Effects of Chronic Ketamine Use on Frontal and Medial Temporal Cognition," *Addictive Behaviors* 38 (2013): 2128–2132, https://doi.org/10.1016/j.addbeh.2013.01.014.

10. J. F. Jhang, Y. H. Hsu, and H. C. Kuo, "Possible Pathophysiology of Ketamine-Related Cystitis and Associated Treatment Strategies," *International Journal of Urology* 22 (2015): 816–825, https://doi.org/10.1111/iju.12841.

11. K. A. Trujillo and C. Y. Heller, "Ketamine Sensitization: Influence of Dose, Environment, Social Isolation and Treatment Interval," *Behavioural Brain Research* 378 (2020): 112271, https://doi.org/10.1016/j.bbr.2019.112271.

12. H. V. Curran and L. Monaghan, "In and Out of the K-hole: A Comparison of the Acute and Residual Effects of Ketamine in Frequent and Infrequent

Ketamine Users," *Addiction* 96 (2001): 749–760, https://doi.org/10.1046/j.1360-0443.2001.96574910.x.
13. R. Narendran, W. G. Frankle, R. Keefe, R. Gil, D. Martinez, M. Slifstein, et al., "Altered Prefrontal Dopaminergic Function in Chronic Recreational Ketamine Users," *American Journal of Psychiatry* 162 (2005): 2352–2359, https://doi.org/10.1176/appi.ajp.162.12.2352.
14. J. L. Vande Voort, R. J. Morgan, S. Kung, K. G. Rasmussen, J. Rico, B. A. Palmer, et al., "Continuation Phase Intravenous Ketamine in Adults with Treatment-Resistant Depression," *Journal of Affective Disorders* 206 (2016): 300–304, https://doi.org/10.1016/j.jad.2016.09.008.
15. A. T. Beck, M. Kovacs, and A. Weissman, "Assessment of Suicidal Intention: The Scale for Suicide Ideation," *Journal of Consulting and Clinical Psychology* 47 (1979): 343–352, https://doi.org/10.1037//0022-006x.47.2.343.
16. J. W. Grimm, B. T. Hope, R. A. Wise, and Y. Shaham, "Neuroadaptation: Incubation of Cocaine Craving after Withdrawal," *Nature* 412 (2001): 141–142, https://doi.org/10.1038/35084134.
17. C. L. Pickens, M. Airavaara, F. Theberge, S. Fanous, B. T. Hope, and Y. Shaham, "Neurobiology of the Incubation of Drug Craving," *Trends in Neuroscience* 34 (2011): 411–420, https://doi.org/10.1016/j.tins.2011.06.001.
18. H. Geoffroy and F. Noble, "BDNF during Withdrawal," *Vitamins & Hormones* 104 (2017): 475–496, https://doi.org/10.1016/bs.vh.2016.10.009.

Chapter 7

1. S. Snelders, C. Kaplan, and T. Pieters, "On Cannabis, Chloral Hydrate, and Career Cycles of Psychotropic Drugs in Medicine," *Bulletin of the History of Medicine* 80 (2006): 95–114, https://doi.org/10.1353/bhm.2006.0041.
2. J. L. Reed, A. C. Nugent, M. L. Furey, J. E. Szczepanik, J. W. Evans, and C. A. Zarate Jr., "Effects of Ketamine on Brain Activity during Emotional Processing: Differential Findings in Depressed versus Healthy Control Participants," *Biological Psychiatry: Cognitive Neuroscience and Neuroimaging* 4 (2019): 610–618, https://doi.org/10.1016/j.bpsc.2019.01.005.
3. M. Spies, M. Klöbl, A. Höflich, A. Hummer, T. Vanicek, P. Michenthaler, et al., "Association between Dynamic Resting-State Functional Connectivity and Ketamine Plasma Levels in Visual Processing Networks," *Scientific Reports* 9 (2019): 11484, https://doi.org/10.1038/s41598-019-46702-x.
4. R. L. Carhart-Harris, M. Bolstridge, J. Rucker, C. M. J. Day, D. Erritzoe, M. Kaelen, et al., "Psilocybin with Psychological Support for Treatment-Resistant Depression: An Open-Label Feasibility Study," *Lancet Psychiatry* 3 (2016): 619–627, https://doi.org/10.1016/s2215-0366(16)30065-7.

5. R. Kraehenmann, K. H. Preller, M. Scheidegger, T. Pokorny, O. G. Bosch, E. Seifritz, et al., "Psilocybin-Induced Decrease in Amygdala Reactivity Correlates with Enhanced Positive Mood in Healthy Volunteers," *Biological Psychiatry* 78 (2015): 572–581, https://doi.org/10.1016/j.biopsych.2014.04.010; L. J. Mertens, M. B. Wall, L. Roseman, L. Demetriou, D. J. Nutt, and R. Carhart-Harris, "Therapeutic Mechanisms of Psilocybin: Changes in Amygdala and Prefrontal Functional Connectivity during Emotional Processing after Psilocybin for Treatment-Resistant Depression," *Journal of Psychopharmacology* 34, no. 2 (2020): 167–180, https://doi.org/10.1177/0269881119895520.

6. S. B. Goldberg, B. T. Pace, C. R. Nicholas, C. L. Raison, and P. R. Hutson, "The Experimental Effects of Psilocybin on Symptoms of Anxiety and Depression: A Meta-analysis," *Psychiatry Research* 284 (2020): 112749, https://doi.org/10.1016/j.psychres.2020.112749.

FURTHER READING

Denomme, N. B. S. "The Domino Effect: Ed Domino's Early Studies of Psychoactive Drugs." *Journal of Psychoactive Drugs* 50 (2018): 298–305.

Jansen, K. L., and R. Darracot-Cankovic. "The Nonmedical Use of Ketamine: A Review of Problem Use and Dependence." *Journal of Psychoactive Drugs* 33 (2001): 151–158.

Mathew, Sanjay J., and Carlos A. Zarate Jr., eds. *Ketamine for Treatment-Resistant Depression: The First Decade of Progress*. New York: Springer, 2016.

Pollan, Michael. *How to Change Your Mind: What the New Science of Psychedelics Teaches Us About Consciousness, Dying, Addiction, Depression, and Transcendence*. New York: Penguin Group Publishing.

INDEX

Academic-industry partnership, 7
Acetylcholine, 51, 56
Adolescent, 22, 61, 65, 129
Aghajanian, George, 87, 106, 109
Allergan, 112
AMPA Receptor, 44–45
Amphetamines, 73–76, 81. *See also* Benzedrine; Dexedrine
Anesthesia, 10, 15, 18–21, 58, 63, 72, 114, 128, 134. *See also* Anesthetic; Subanesthetic
Anesthetic, 8–11,17–20, 24, 27, 49–50, 58–64, 91–92, 96–97, 128, 134, 151
Antidepressant drug discovery, 1–2, 78–81
Antidepressant drugs. *See* Amphetamines; Opiates, opioids, and their receptors; SSRI; Tricyclic antidepressants
Antipsychotics, 2, 24, 26, 73, 78–79, 134. *See also* Chlorpromazine (thorazine)
Anxiety, 74–75
Arketamine 15, 97, 99, 116, 132
Astra, 82
Avicenna (Ibn Sina), 70

Barbiturates, 10, 18, 75, 76
BDNF (brain-derived neurotrophic factor), 89–90, 106–107, 109, 112, 113, 138, 157
Benzedrine, 73–74
"Black box" warning, xi

Carter-Wallace, 74, 75, 77
Catalepsy, 7, 8
CDC (Centers for Disease Control and Prevention), 66
Charney, Dennis, 87, 94–95
China, 22, 133
Chirality, 11–15
Chlorpromazine (thorazine), 24, 73, 78–79
Chronic pain management, 21, 59
Ciba-Geigy, 17
Club drug, 21, 22
Cognitive deficits, 61–63, 129
COMPASS Pathways, 151

DEA (Drug Enforcement Administration), 151
Delgado, Pedro, 87
Depression *See also* Major depressive disorder
  animal models, 84–86, 105, 146
  clinical features, 65–68
  monoamine hypothesis, 81–89
  nonpharmacologic therapies, 68
Dexedrine, 73, 75, 76
Diagnostic and Statistical Manual of Mental Disorders, 65
Dirty drug, 43, 51, 52, 158
Disinhibition, 49–50, 106–108
Dissociative, 22, 117, 134
Domino, Edward F., 8–11
Dopamine, 53–55, 61, 64, 136
DSM, 65

Duloxetine (Cymbalta), 80
Duman, Ron, 106

Ecstasy, 149
Electroconvulsive therapy (ECT), 72–73, 117–119
Eli Lilly, 83
Esketamine (Spravato), 15, 70, 97–100, 116, 121–122, 124–128, 130–132, 135, 138, 142–144
Estrogen, 54, 115
Excitatory-inhibitory balance, 64

Fluoxetin. *See* Prozac
Food and Drug Administration (FDA), xi, 5, 11, 15, 21, 27, 78–79, 83, 95, 99, 121–124, 126, 128, 150–151,158–159

Geigy, 3, 78, 79
Glia, 57–58, 62, 115
Glutamate, 46–51, 56–58, 93, 106–112
Gordon, Joshua, xi

Heninger, George, 87
Hoffmann-La Roche, 74
Hofman, Albert, 3
Hong Kong, 22, 133

Imipramine (Tofranin), 3, 78, 79
Inflammation, 114–115
Iproniazid, 78
Isoniazid, 2

Janssen, 95, 99, 122
Javitt, Daniel, 26
Johnson & Johnson, 95, 97, 98, 99, 122, 125, 126, 127, 138

K-hole, 22, 63
K-land, 22
Kline, Nathan F, 26, 78
Krystal, John, 26–27, 91, 93–95, 99, 155
Kuhn, Ronald, 79

Laudanum, 70–72
LSD, 3, 53, 149
Luby, Elliot, 10, 24

Maddox, Victor, 1, 7
Major depressive disorder (MDD), 65, 68, 90, 94, 114, 122, 125
Malaysia, 22, 133
Manji, Husseini, 95
MAO inhibitor, 81, 83, 86
McEwen, Bruce, 89, 108
Membrane voltage, 35–36, 45
Meprobamate (Deprol), 74
Metabolites of ketamine, 58–59, 109
Miltown (Dexamyl), 74, 75, 77
Monoamine oxidase (MAO), 80–83, 86
Monteggia, Lisa, 108–109
Morphine, 72
Mount Sinai School of Medicine, 95

Naltrexone (Vivitrol, ReVia), 117
Neuroinflammatory mechanisms, 114–115
Neurons, 34–57, 89, 102, 105–108
Neuropharmacology, 8
Neuropsychopharmacology, 1
Neuroscience, 31, 60, 73, 86, 95, 101, 127, 146
Neurotransmitter, 37–46, 51, 53, 56

NIH (National Institutes of Health), 84, 94, 95
NIMH (National Institute of Mental Health), 94, 95
Nitrazine, 2
NMDA receptor, 44–49, 57, 93, 122–127, 145
Noradrenaline, 79–80, 86
Novartis, 3

OCD (obsessive-compulsive disorder), 3
Off-label use, 21, 24, 95, 128, 139
Opiates, opioids, and their receptors, 21, 53, 60, 70–72, 90, 116–117. *See also* Laudanum; Morphine; Naltrexone

Pain, 7, 11, 18, 21, 53, 62
Parke-Davis, 1, 5–11
Paxil, 83
PCP (phencyclidine), 1, 7–11, 24–27, 106
Pediatric, 18
Peptide, 37, 53
Pharmaceutical companies. *See* Allergan; Astra; Carter-Wallace; COMPASS Pathways; Eli Lilly; Geigy; Hoffman-La Roche; Janssen; Johnson & Johnson; Parke-Davis; Smith Kline and French; Usona; Wyatt
Polymorphism, 59
Prozac (fluoxetine), 68, 69, 81, 83–84,101, 104, 107
Psilocybin, 149–152
Psychedelic, 149. *See also* LSD; Psilocybin
Psychosis, 2, 63, 79, 81, 93, 97, 99, 128, 134
Psychotic, 15, 18, 23, 26, 70

Rapastinel, 112, 145
Receptor, 24, 37–57, 64, 79–80, 82, 93, 101–118, 145
Rhesus monkeys, 8, 10

Sandoz, 3
Sapolsky, Robert, 89, 108
Schizophrenia, 10, 24, 26–29, 61, 63, 64, 73, 78, 79, 90, 91, 93–94
Sedative, 59, 74, 75, 76, 77
Seige, Max, 141
Seige cycle, 141,144
Sernyl, 10
Serotonin, 37, 53–55, 79–83, 86–88, 101
Smith Kline and French (SKF), 73, 75
SNRI (serotonin-norepinephrine reuptake inhibitor), 79–80, 84, 86
Spravato, 99, 121–127
SSRI (selective serotonin reuptake inhibitor), 81–87, 89, 101, 105, 114, 146
Subanesthetic, 27, 60, 61, 62, 63, 91, 94, 102, 129, 134
Suicide, 22, 66, 100, 124–125, 136–139, 141, 152
Synapse, 34–40, 44–45

Tolerance, xi, 62, 133, 134, 135, 144
Tranquilizers, 74
TRD (treatment-resistant depression), 114–115, 117, 122–124, 126, 160

Tricyclic antidepressants, 78–81, 146
Tryptophan, 87–88
Tuberculosis (TB), 2, 4, 78, 80
Turner, D. M., 23

Ulcerative cystitis, 23, 64, 133
Usona, 151

VA (US Department of Veterans Affairs), 26, 27, 91, 94, 126, 127
Valium, 59, 74
Veterinary, 20, 21, 60
Vietnam War, 17

Wayne State University, 1,1 0, 11
Witczak, Kim, 122, 124
Wyatt, 74

Yale, 26, 86, 87, 91, 94, 95, 106, 155

Zarate, Carlos, 95
Zimelidine (Zelmid), 82

The MIT Press Essential Knowledge Series

AI Ethics, Mark Coeckelbergh
Algorithms, Panos Louridas
Annotation, Remi H. Kalir and Antero Garcia
Anticorruption, Robert I. Rotberg
Auctions, Timothy P. Hubbard and Harry J. Paarsch
Behavioral Insights, Michael Hallsworth and Elspeth Kirkman
The Book, Amaranth Borsuk
Carbon Capture, Howard J. Herzog
Citizenship, Dimitry Kochenov
Cloud Computing, Nayan B. Ruparelia
Collaborative Society, Dariusz Jemielniak and Aleksandra Przegalinska
Computational Thinking, Peter J. Denning and Matti Tedre
Computing: A Concise History, Paul E. Ceruzzi
The Conscious Mind, Zoltan E. Torey
Contraception: A Concise History, Donna J. Drucker
Critical Thinking, Jonathan Haber
Crowdsourcing, Daren C. Brabham
Cynicism, Ansgar Allen
Data Science, John D. Kelleher and Brendan Tierney
Deep Learning, John D. Kelleher
Extraterrestrials, Wade Roush
Extremism, J. M. Berger
Fake Photos, Hany Farid
fMRI, Peter A. Bandettini
Food, Fabio Parasecoli
Free Will, Mark Balaguer
The Future, Nick Montfort
GPS, Paul E. Ceruzzi
Haptics, Lynette A. Jones
Hate Speech, Caitlin Ring Carlson
Information and Society, Michael Buckland
Information and the Modern Corporation, James W. Cortada
Intellectual Property Strategy, John Palfrey
The Internet of Things, Samuel Greengard
Irony and Sarcasm, Roger Kreuz
Ketamine, Bita Moghaddam
Machine Learning: The New AI, Ethem Alpaydín

Machine Translation, Thierry Poibeau
Macroeconomics, Felipe Larraín B.
Memes in Digital Culture, Limor Shifman
Metadata, Jeffrey Pomerantz
The Mind–Body Problem, Jonathan Westphal
MOOCs, Jonathan Haber
Neuroplasticity, Moheb Costandi
Nihilism, Nolen Gertz
Open Access, Peter Suber
Paradox, Margaret Cuonzo
Phenomenology, Chad Engelland
Post-Truth, Lee McIntyre
Quantum Entanglement, Jed Brody
Recommendation Engines, Michael Schrage
Recycling, Finn Arne Jørgensen
Robots, John Jordan
School Choice, David R. Garcia
Science Fiction, Sherryl Vint
Self-Tracking, Gina Neff and Dawn Nafus
Sexual Consent, Milena Popova
Smart Cities, Germaine R. Halegoua
Spaceflight: A Concise History, Michael J. Neufeld
Spatial Computing, Shashi Shekhar and Pamela Vold
Sustainability, Kent E. Portney
Synesthesia, Richard E. Cytowic
The Technological Singularity, Murray Shanahan
3D Printing, John Jordan
Understanding Beliefs, Nils J. Nilsson
Virtual Reality, Samuel Greengard
Visual Culture, Alexis L. Boylan
Waves, Frederic Raichlen

BITA MOGHADDAM is a neuroscientist and the author of nearly 150 scientific papers, including original and influential research related to the mechanism of action of ketamine. Her work has been cited over twenty thousand times and has been continuously funded by the National Institutes of Health since 1991. She is currently the Ruth Matarazzo Professor of Behavioral Neuroscience at Oregon Health and Science University (OHSU). She was a professor of psychiatry and neurobiology at Yale and professor of neuroscience at the University of Pittsburgh before joining OHSU in 2017.